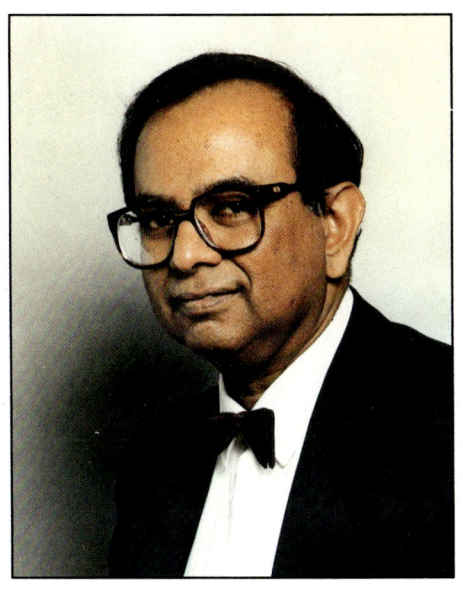

AUTHOR:
Dr. Munsif Meeran, MBBS, DRCOG, Licentiate in Acupuncture, FRSM
Formerly Director Zambia Flying Doctor Service
Consultant Obstetrician and Gynaecologist Libya
President Red Cross Society Zambia
Presently: Director of Studies, Marina Academy and Supplies International,
Member British Medical Acupuncture Society.
Consultant to F.D.S. Programmes
Member British Medical Laser Association
Director and Founder Member London Medical Acupuncture Auricular Therapy Society (L.M.A.S. Ltd)

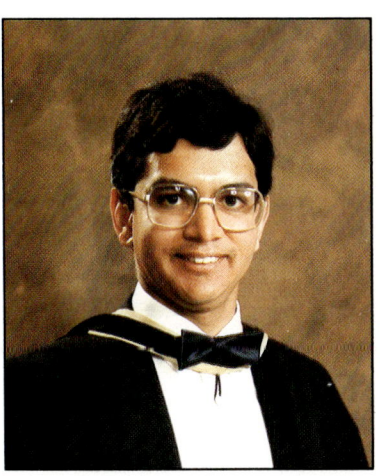

CO-AUTHOR:
Dr. Karim Meeran, B.Sc. (Hons.) MBBS (Hons.)
Lecturer Marina Academy and Supplies International
Associate Member British Medical Acupuncture Society.
Member London Medical Acupuncture Auricular Therapy Society (L.M.A.S. Ltd)

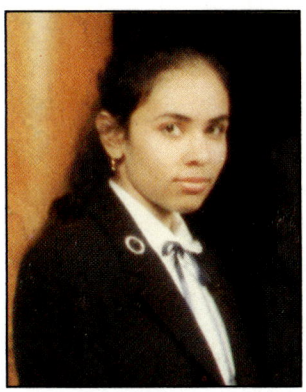

COMPILED BY:
Miss Marina Aida Meeran, Undergraduate King's College London
Demonstrator Marina Academy and Supplies International.

to
Ummu
with love

Meeran's Colour Atlas of Acupuncture Auricular Therapy
and Lasers
First Published in 1990 by
© Marina Academy Publishers international

All rights reserved. No part of this publication may be reproduced, stored in a retrieval system, or transmitted in any form or by any means, electronic, mechanical, photocopying, recording or otherwise, without the prior permission of the publishers.
Marina Academy Publishers International 30, Lismore Road, South Croydon, England CR2 7QA
Printed in Hong Kong.

ISBN 1 870634 02 0

FOREWORD
by
Dr. M. H. M. Hamza, M.B., F.R.C.P., D.C.H.

I had the rare privilege to visit China during the height of the Cultural Revolution, and I had the rarer opportunity to visit hospitals, in the larger cities of that great country, and to observe, how the ancient art and science of acupuncture and other forms of traditional Chinese medicine is taught and practised. However, books on the subject, in English, I found, hard to come by. They were literally non existent. Hopefully, this anomaly has been reversed, and to satisfy the demands of an ever increasing clientele of students and practitioners of acupuncture, there are, now, readily available, a glut of books and charts. Nevertheless, many of the books, are repetitive, laborious, confusing, involved and enshrouded in mystique and folklore!!!

This elegantly produced atlas on acupuncture and auriculotherapy, by Dr. Munsif Meeran is clear, concise, and easy to understand. The excellent colour pictures are brilliant, bright and the illustrations are a sheer delight. This Atlas, carries with it, without having to wade through voluminous and involved books on the subject, the ingredients, for an in-depth grasp and appreciation of the basic principles of the science and art of acupuncture. This Atlas, I firmly believe, will meet the felt needs of students and practitioners alike.

Dr. Munsif Meeran, is an excellent teacher, and as such, has maintained the belief, that communicating exciting ideas on a subject is more important than the mere acquistion of detailed facts. He has, therefore, jettisoned much of the small print stuff. However, he has included a number of topics which I found hand-rubbingly irresistable. There are tidbits, too, which enliven, excite, and add a unique feel and flavour to the Atlas, which will, surely, be recognised and appreciated by those genuinely interested in the subject.

As a starting point, for all those interested in the fascinating subject of the practice of acupuncture and auriculotherapy Dr. Meeran's Atlas cannot be bettered. The clarity of the Atlas spares the reader from contending with fanciful concepts and folklore. Far from being another book, to gather dust on the shelves, this exciting Atlas will be regularly consulted, by all interested in acupuncture and auriculotherapy. Its refreshingly direct approach, to sets of problems guarantees Dr. Meeran's Atlas to become a classic on the subject of acupuncture and auriculotherapy.

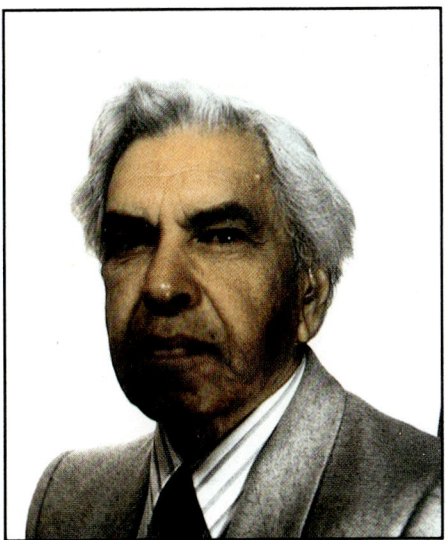

Dr. M. H. M. Hamza

Formerly Consultant Paediatrician, Lady Ridgeway Childrens Hospital, Colombo.
Professor of Paediatrics World Health Organisation (WHO).
Senior Lecturer, Institute of Child Health, University of London.
Hon. Consultant, Hospital for Sick Children, Great Ormond Street, London.
Presently Visiting Lecturer Swiss Tropical Institute Basel, Switzerland.
Member British Medical Acupuncture Society.
Vice-Patron and Founder Member London Medical Acupuncture Auricular Therapy Society (L.M.A.S. Ltd)

PREFACE

This Atlas has been produced for those doctors, acupuncturists, students and all those interested in practising acupuncture and auricular therapy as a result of many requests. It gives at a glance an understanding of Meridians and Pathways and Acupuncture Points and their Locations — It opens up horizons to auricular therapy in the ear.

This Atlas is a ready-reckoner and gives formulae or prescriptions for ailments at a glance and gives accurately the basis of Acupuncture, Auricular and Laser therapy.

The systems discussed and described in the Atlas are stated under Contents.

The Authors wish to thank:

Shamim Nurbhai for the painstaking efforts for the arrangements and for the editing of the relevant scripts of the various sections of this Atlas.

Cassim Humzah for the help in taking the photgraphs, and
Amin Ismail for photographs, illustrations and for designing the cover and Nihara Ismail for her suggestions.

Jack Berry(Manager) and Karen O'Brien of UDO Croydon for their co-operation, patience and helping me with the production of this Atlas.

Dr. M. H. M. Hamza, MB, FRCP, DCH
Formerly Professor of Paediatrics World Health Organisation (WHO)
Presently Visiting Lecturer Swiss Tropical Institute, Basle, Switzerland; Member British Medical Acupuncture Society.
for encouraging and persuading me (the author) to produce this Atlas as he felt this production will be very useful to all interested in Acupuncture.

Special thanks to Mr. Trevor Peace for his expertise in the layout of this Atlas, the Author and Co-Author know that without Mr. Peace's dedication that this Atlas would not have become a reality.

Nelson Press Co. Ltd. in the Isle of Man for Typesetting and Camera ready Artwork.
Camerawork, Colour Separation and Planning by Moody Graphics Int., 4-8 Emerson St., London SE1 9DU. Tel: 01-928 8486
Nasreen Bawa - Management Accountant, Cambridge - for proof reading the text of this Atlas.

AUTHOR:
Dr. Munsif Meeran, MBBS, DRCOG Licentiate in Acupuncture, FRSM,
Formerly: Director Zambia Flying Doctor Service,
Consultant Obstetrician and Gynaecologist Libya
President Red Cross Society, Zambia,
Presently: Director of Studies, Marina Academy and Supplies International,
Member British Medical Acupuncture Society,
Consultant to F.D.S. Programmes.
Member British Medical Laser Association
Founder Member London Medical Acupuncture Auricular Therapy Society (L.M.A.S. Ltd)

CO-AUTHOR:
Dr. Karim Meeran, B.Sc. (Hons.), MBBS (Hons.),
Lecturer Marina Academy and Supplies International,
Associate Member British Medical Acupuncture Society.
Member London Medical Acupuncture Auricular Therapy Society (L.M.A.S. Ltd)

COMPILED BY:
Miss Marina Aida Meeran, Undergraduate King's College, London,
Demonstrator Marina Academy and Supplies International,

PUBLISHERS:
Marina Academy and Supplies International
30-32 Lismore Road
South Croydon
Surrey CR2 7QA
United Kingdom

SOLE DISTRIBUTORS:

MARINA ACADEMY INTERNATIONAL
30 Lismore Road,
South Croydon, CR2 7QA
UNITED KINGDOM
Fax: 01 667-9522

THE MEERAN COLOUR ATLAS OF ACUPUNCTURE, AURICULAR THERAPY AND LASER THERAPY

CONTENTS

Introduction
Yin-yang, five elements, needles and acupunctoscope.
Classical system of meridians in body acupuncture.
The 12 ordinary and the 2 extra ordinary meridians showing important acupuncture points used.

1. The Anatomy of the Skeletal system, Joints and Muscles 1
2. Needles and Electro Acupuncture 13
3. The twelve ordinary meridians 19
4. The two extra-ordinary meridians and Meeran's Laws for Meridians 33
5. Pain Pathway & Gate Control theory of Melzack & Wall 37
6. Laser therapy: Its uses in acupuncture and auriculotherapy 41
7. Ear Acupuncture 47
    (a) Anatomy
    (b) Acupuncture Points
    (c) Specific Zones
    (d) Cartography of the Ear including ear geometry
8. Assessment and Management 55
9. Treatment of pain and disease 59
    (a) Migraine
    (b) Facial Pain
    (c) Lower limb and foot
10. Orthopaedics and Rheumatology 63
    (a) Cervical Pain and Cervical Spondylosis
    (b) Lumbo-Sacral pain and back aches
    (c) Arthritis of the hip and knee
    (d) Arthritis of the Shoulder
    (e) Carpal Tunnel Syndrome
11. Neurology 73
    (a) Bell's Palsy
    (b) Trigeminal Neuralgia and Facial pain
    (c) Menieres Syndrome
    (d) Acupuncture sympathectomy for peripheral vascular disease
12. Anti-Smoking and Obesity programmes 77
13. Sinusitis, Headaches and Dermatology 81
    (a) Acne
    (b) Cosmetic Acupuncture
    (c) Alopecia
14. Painless Childbirth 85

CONTENTS - Continued

15. Psycho-Somatics ... 91
    (a) Nervous Tension Points
    (b) Anxiety, Phobias and Depression

16. Endocrinology ... 95
    (a) Hormones controlling Breast development and function
    (b) Anatomy of the Breast
    (c) Lactation
    (d) Cosmetic Acupuncture for Breast enlargement
    (e) Hypercalcaemia-calcitonin point in auricle and treatment of bone pain

17. Subfertility ... 101

18. Psycho-Sexual Problems ... 105
    (a) Impotence
    (b) Frigidity
    (c) Dyspareunia

19. Nose, Hand and Foot Acupuncture ... 109

20. Scalp or Head Acupuncture ... 113

21. Miscellaneous Facts and Treatments ... 119

22. Starting an Acupuncture Clinic ... 123
    (a) Equipment
    (b) Needles - Body and Ear Needles
    (c) Lasers etc.

23. Treatment of Drug Addicts and Alcoholics ... 127
    (a) The use of disposable needles

Index ... 136

*"From inability to leave well alone;
From too much zeal for what is new and
    contempt for what is old;
From putting knowledge before wisdom.
science before art, cleverness before commonsense;
From treating patients as cases; and
From making the cure of a disease more
    grievous than its endurance,
Good Lord, deliver us."*

Sir Robert Hutchison (1871 - 1960)

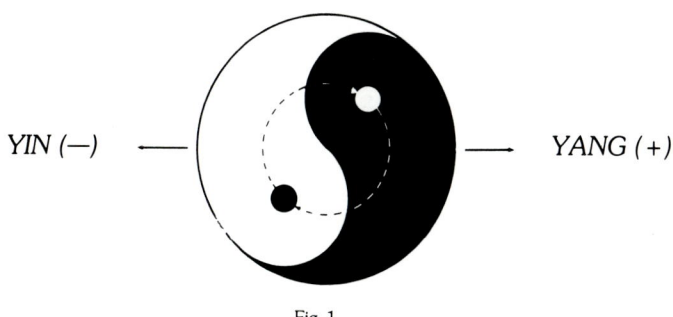

Fig. 1

THE CHINESE MONAD

Yin and Yang are forces which, according to Chinese philosophy control the various manifestations in the universe. Yang is the positive pole and Yin is the negative pole. The diagram illustrates a very important principle which the Chinese knew more than 6,000 years ago. The arrows indicate the forces and if the Yin and Yang are not balanced, the body does not function properly and this results in disease. It must be emphasised that even though the words Yin and Yang may look abstract to the reader, they are not as complex as they seem. To put it simply, YIN means hypo-function and the word YANG means hyper-function. This indicates that the organ or bowel is not in balance and would explain the phenomenon of disease.

THE FIVE ELEMENT SYSTEM

The Five-element System represents the five elements — fire, earth, metal, water and wood (abbrev. F.E.M.W.W.). From the diagram it is clear that there are twelve representations (organs and bowels) and each of these representations has its own meridian which is called the **ordinary** meridians as opposed to the **extraordinary** meridians.

There are approximately 800-1,000 acupuncture points in the body. At the outset it must be emphasised that it is not essential to know all these points. Approximately 365 of these points belong to the 12 Ordinary Meridians plus the Governor Vessel and Conception Vessel as set out below:—

Lung	11	Liver	14
Colon	20	Pericardium	9
Stomach	45	Three-heater	23
Spleen	21	Small Intestine	21
Heart	9	Governor Vessel	28
Kidney	27	Conception Vessel	24
Gall Bladder	44	Urinary Bladder	67*

*This meridian has the most number of points.

YIN Organs:
Heart (H), Pericardium (P), Kidney (KI), Liver (LI), Spleen (SP), Lung (LU).

YANG Organs:
Stomach (ST), Three Heater (TH), Gall Bladder (GB), Bladder (BL), Colon (CO), Small Intestine (SI),

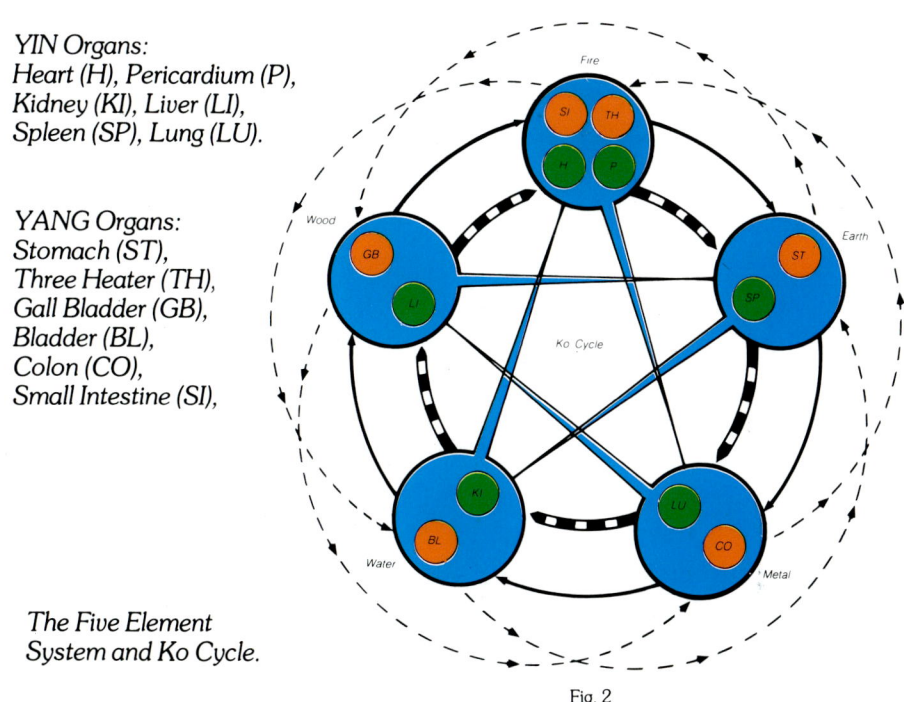

The Five Element System and Ko Cycle.

Fig. 2

THE 12 ORDINARY MERIDIANS AND THE 2 EXTRA-ORDINARY MERIDIANS

1. THE LUNG MERIDIAN has a descending flow of energy running from the top of the chest along the inside of the arm to the outside of the thumb. It is bilaterally represented and has 11 POINTS.

2. THE COLON MERIDIAN has an ascending flow of energy running from the tip of the index finger of the hand to the side of the nose. It is bilaterally represented and has 20 POINTS.

3. THE STOMACH MERIDIAN has a descending flow of energy starting from the head to the foot. It is bilaterally represented and has 45 POINTS.

4. THE SPLEEN MERIDIAN has an ascending flow of energy running from the foot upward to the chest. It is bilaterally represented and has 21 POINTS.

5. THE HEART MERIDIAN has a descending flow of energy starting from the chest to the hand. It is bilaterally represented and has 9 POINTS.

6. THE SMALL INTESTINE MERIDIAN has an ascending flow of energy running from the hand to the head and has 19 POINTS.

7. THE BLADDER MERIDIAN has a descending flow of energy from the head downward to the foot. It is bilaterally represented and has 67 POINTS.

8. THE KIDNEY MERIDIAN has an ascending flow of energy running from the foot to the chest. It is bilaterally represented and has 27 POINTS.

9. THE HEART CONSTRICTOR MERIDIAN has a descending flow of energy commencing from the chest to the hand. It is bilaterally represented with 9 POINTS.

10. THE TRIPLE HEATER MERIDIAN has an ascending flow of energy running from the hand up to the head. It is bilaterally represented and has 23 POINTS.

11. THE GALL BLADDER MERIDIAN has a descending flow of energy running from the chest to the foot. It is bilaterally reperesented and has 44 POINTS.

12. THE LIVER MERIDIAN has an ascending flow of energy starting from the foot upwards to the chest. It is bilaterally represented and has 14 POINTS.

13. THE GOVERNOR VESSEL has an ascending flow of energy from the tip of the coccyx. It is a midline vessel on the dorsal aspect and crosses the middle of the scalp, tip of the nose and ends in the philtrum of the upper lip, on the mucosal side. It has 28 POINTS.

14. THE CONCEPTION VESSEL is a single vessel and ascends from the perineum, symphysis pubis, umbilicus and ends at the lower border of the lip. It has 24 POINTS.

Illustration of Acupuncture Points

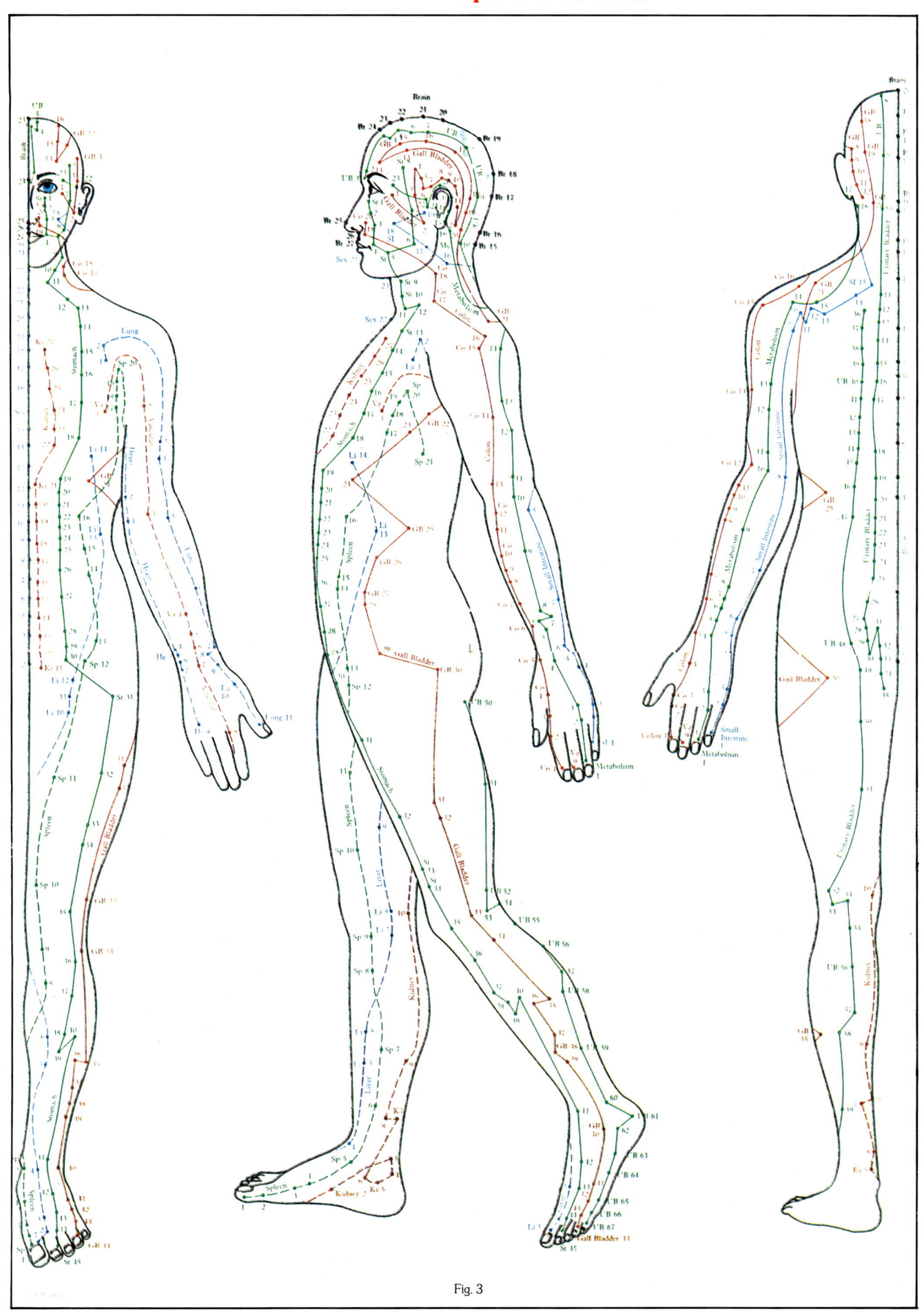

Fig. 3

The Skeletal System

Joints

Muscular System

THE SKELETAL SYSTEM

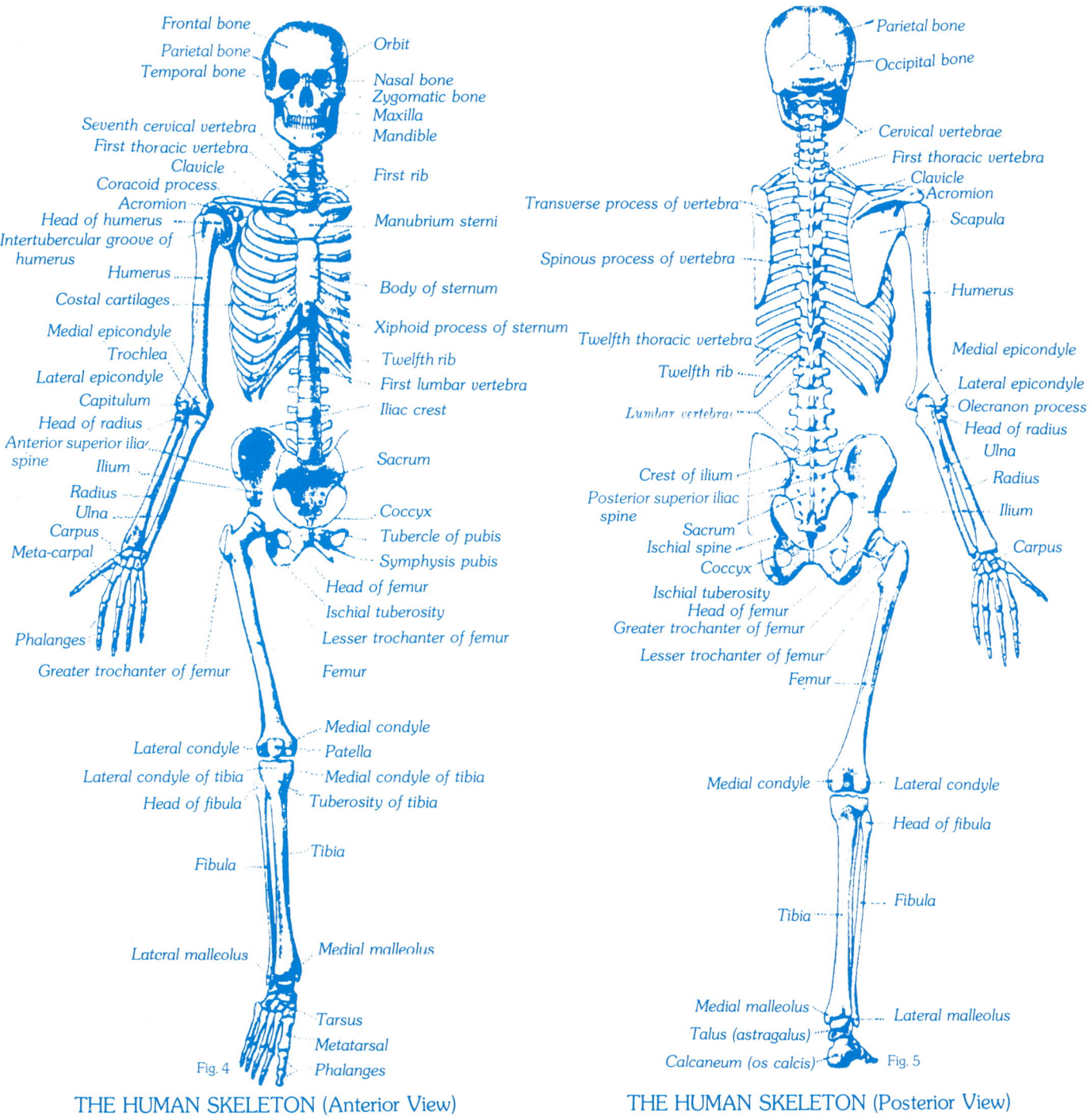

THE HUMAN SKELETON (Anterior View)   THE HUMAN SKELETON (Posterior View)

with courtesy and kind permission of Faber and Faber Ltd. London

CRANIUM OR SKULL

8 bones form the skull. They are:
1 frontal bone, forms the forehead, 2 parietal bones form the top and side of the skull, 1 occipital bone is posterior, 2 temporal bones form the sides of the skull, 1 sphenoid bone forms the greater part of the base of the skull.

BONES OF THE SPINE

33 bones form the spine. 24 true vertebrae are separated by intervertebral discs which allows some movement between the vertebrae. The spine is divided into:
Cervical spine with 7 cervical vertabrae like in all mammals, 12 thoracic or dorsal, 5 lumbar, the sacrum and coccyx.

BONES OF THE THORAX

There are 12 thoracic vertebrae with 12 pairs of ribs which form the sides of the chest. 7 pairs are true ribs, 5 are false ribs and of the 5 two are floating ribs.
The sternum is formed of the manubrium, body and xiphoid process.

BONES OF THE UPPER AND LOWER LIMBS

As shown above.

JOINTS

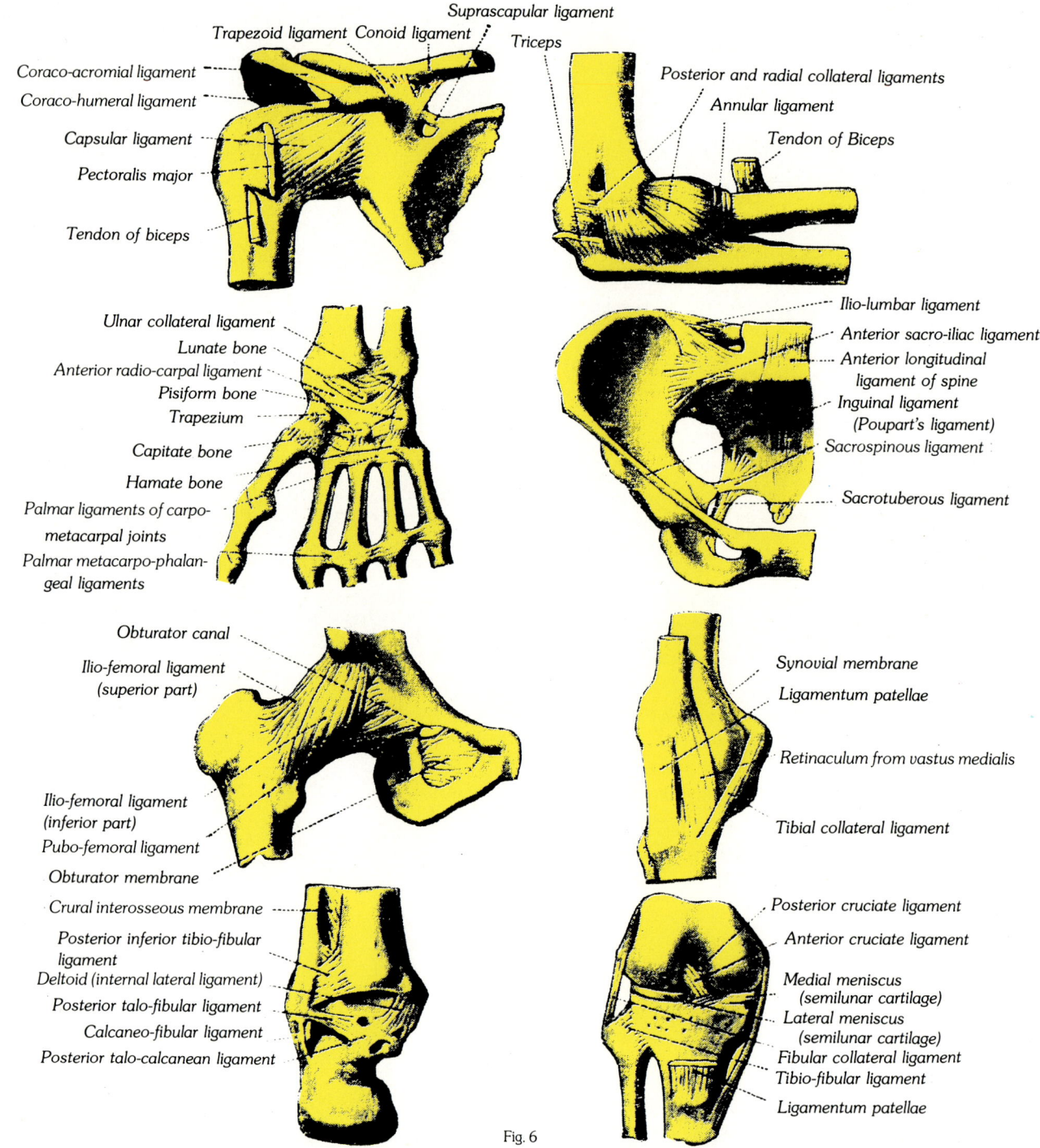

Fig. 6

With courtesy and kind permission of Faber and Faber Ltd. London

JOINTS

Joints are formed where bones articulate with one another. Joints are classified as:—

1. Sutural Joints
2. Primary Cartilaginous Joints, e.g. epiphysis, costo-chondral joint.
   In the above two no movements are possible.
3. Secondary cartilaginous joints, e.g. inter-vertebral discs.
4. Synovial joints. These allow free movement:
   (a) Ball and Socket Joint — hip and shoulder joints.
   (b) Hinge Joints — knee and elbow joints, the superior radio-ulnar joint and (the atlanto-axial joint - pivot joint).
   (c) Condyloid Joints — wrist joint and the metacarpal phalangeal joints.

MUSCULAR SYSTEM

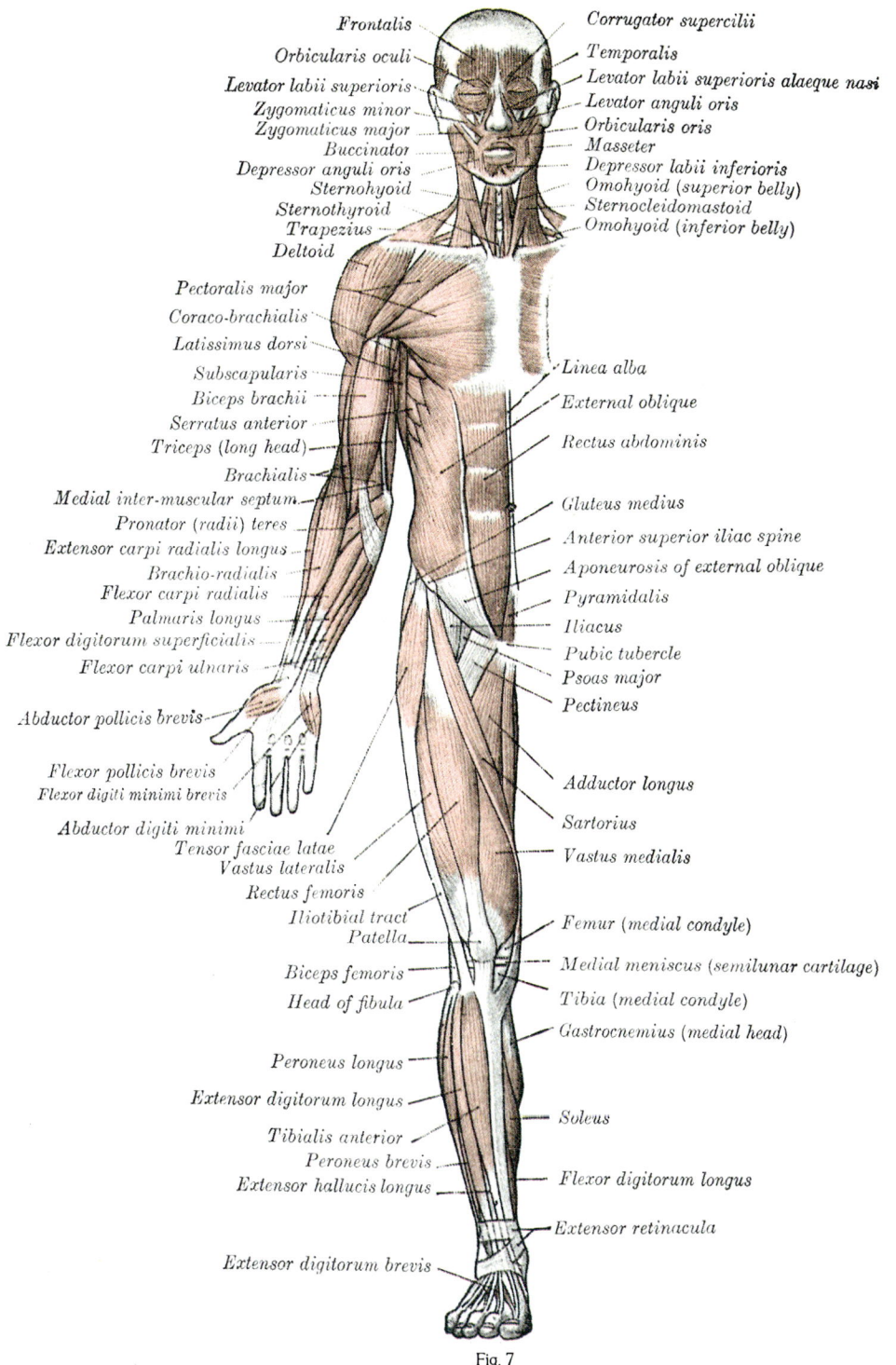

Fig. 7

THE MUSCLES OF THE BODY (Anterior View)

with courtesy and kind permission of Faber and Faber Ltd., London

MUSCLES

The muscles as shown above consist of superficial and deep muscles. These muscles must be known by all acupuncturists as needling of the points will be given as landmarks for the various diseases later in the Atlas in relation to the muscles.

The muscles mass is not just concerned with locomotion but it assists in the circulation of blood and protects and confines the visceral organs. It also provides the main shaping of the human form. A detailed knowledge of myology is of vital importance to acupuncturists because, having established the surface anatomy and exact location of an organ, they must plan the exact route in needling with minimum risk to the patient. On this page are the principal muscles of the anterior aspects of the body.

MUSCULAR SYSTEM

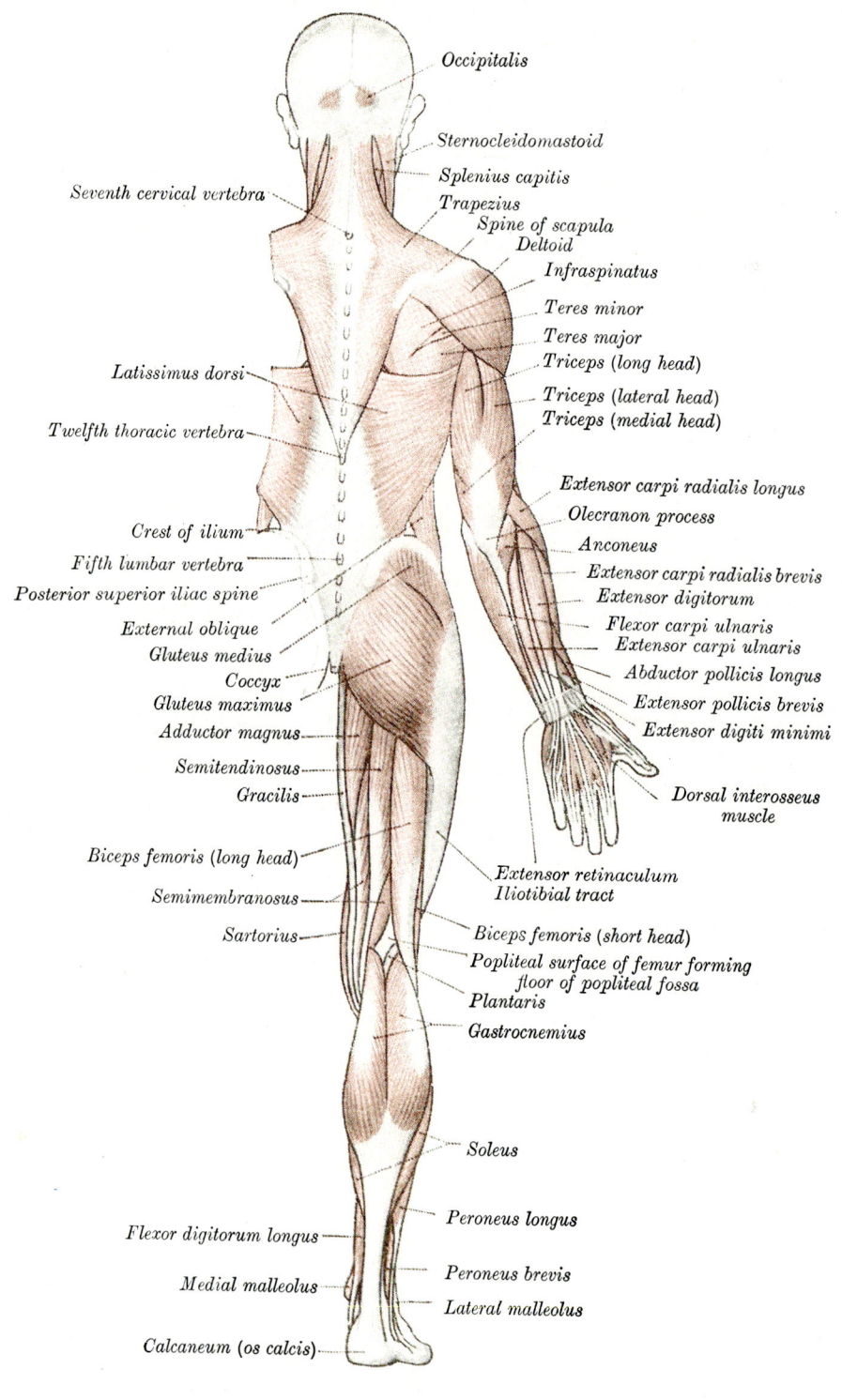

Fig. 8

THE MUSCLES OF THE BODY (Posterior View)

With courtesy and kind permission of Faber and Faber Ltd. London

In the posterior aspect are represented the Governor, Bladder Meridian etc.
> Bladder 11 is at Thoracic spine 1 level.
>
> Bladder 21 is at Thoracic spine 12 level.
>
> Bladder 50 is at midpoint of lower border of Gluteus Maximus.

The most prominent spine is cervical 7 - referred to as Vertebra Prominens and all levels - Anatomically are taken from this level.

MUSCULAR SYSTEM

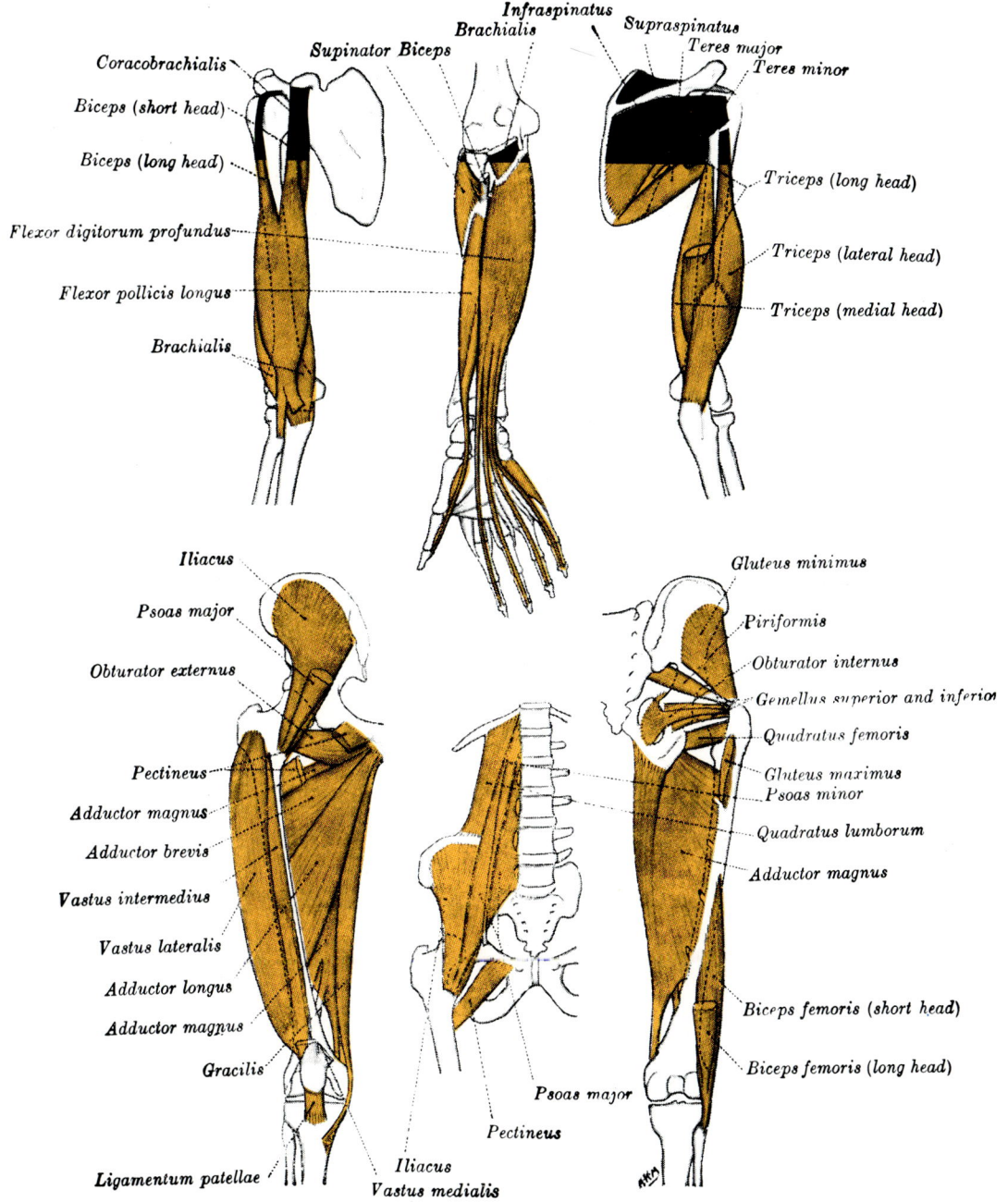

Fig. 9

DEEP MUSCLES

With courtesy and kind permission of Faber and Faber Ltd. London.

THE DEEP MUSCLES

When needles of 1 inch or more are used the Acupuncturist must know exactly what muscles and structures are pierced.

Example:— In the back of the knee in the Popliteal Crease is bladder 54 and this point is often used for backache and sciatica. The Popliteal artery can be felt here - knowledge of deeper muscles must be known, refer standard text books in Anatomy.

Needles and Electro - Acupuncture

1. **Needles and Moxibustion**

2. **Electronic Acupunctoscope - WQ 100**

3. **Electro-Acupuncture**

4. **Advantages of Electro-Acupuncture**

5. **The connection of Electrodes**

ELECTRO - ACUPUNCTURE

The Author and Co-Author are of the opinion that the best machines to use for Electro-Acupuncture are:—

1. WQ 100 Electro-Acupunctoscope
2. IC - 1107 Electro-Acupunctoscope

Other Acupunctoscopes are useful and this may not be the opinion of other Acupuncturists. But in all Patients demonstrated in this Atlas - the WQ 100 or IC - 1107 Electro-Acupunctoscope were used with very good results.

NEEDLES AND MOXIBUSTION

The practice of acupuncture consists of either stimulating or dispersing the flow of energy in the body by inserting needles at specific points on the surface of the skin. A related technique, using heat, or thermal therapy, instead of needles is moxibustion.

The standard filiform needle is made of silver, gold, molybdenum, steel or platinum — the metal used depends on the illness being treated. Unlike a sewing needle it has no eye, but instead a gripping area called the handle. This is joined by the needle root to the body which tapers to a very fine tip. A frequently used needle length is 13mm (½ inch), though some can be 150mm long. They are also of variable thickness: from gauge 34 (0.22mm) to gauge 26 (0.45mm). Not surprisingly these needles can be inserted almost painlessly — with minimum or no discomfort to the patient.

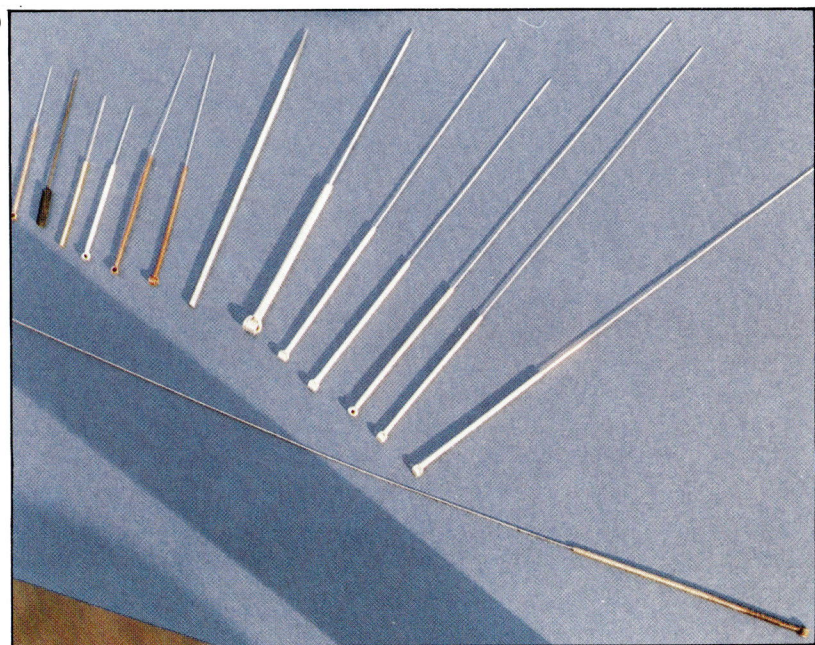

Fig. 10

ACUPUNCTURE NEEDLES. ½" - 6" Metal, Steel, Silver, Molybdenum, Gold. Gauge 32-36 (0.18mm).

Besides the basic filiform needle there is the plum blossom needle — comprising a ring of seven fine needles mounted on one head; the prismatic needle — used for blood letting; the three edged needle; and a range of small needles used specifically for ear acupuncture. The latter are made of gold, silver or steel and can be left in an acupuncture point for two or three weeks.

ELECTROACUPUNCTURE

We have looked at the basics of acupuncture, including what is involved in the process of needling and why it can cure pain and disease. A logical step on from traditional therapy is electroacupuncture, a relatively new healing technique, combining the principles of traditional needling with the advantages of modern technology. In fact nowadays it is normally used instead of manual needling; the only exceptions are a few types of ear therapy.

How is it that in the space of a few decades electroacupuncture has all but ousted its manual counterpart of 6,000 years standing? There are two main reasons: electro-acupuncture is far less cumbersome and slow, and more importantly it gives far better results.

We have learnt that if traditional treatment is to be successful the needles must be inserted in exactly the right place,

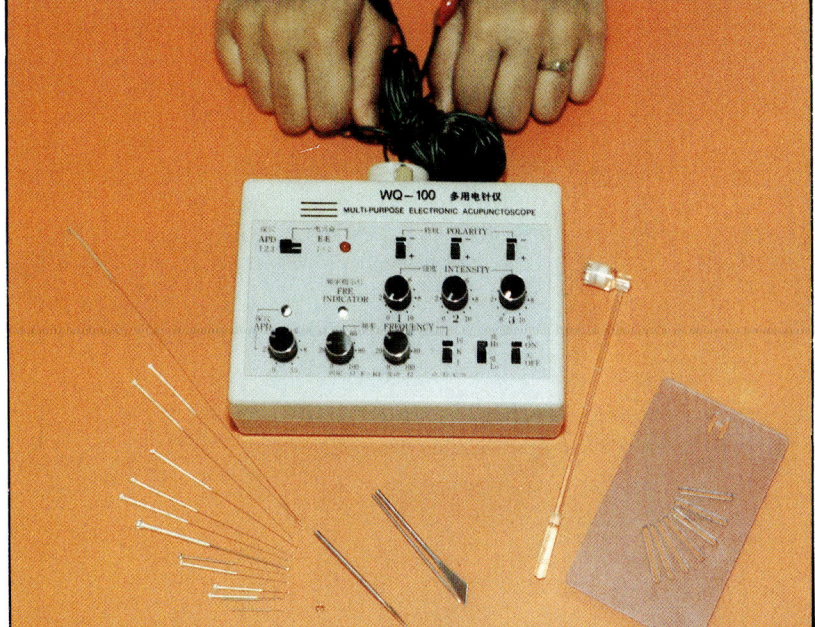

Fig. 11

NEEDLES. WQ-100 Electronic Acupunctoscope, seven star needle and anti-tobacco protractor for 10 needle technique of Nogier.

there is no room for slight error. Once in the correct position the needle must be manipulated by hand; the doctor has to twist it to and fro for anything up to 40 minutes. Even for the simplest of conditions like migraine at least eight needles are used and, though unusual, 20 sessions may be necessary per course of treatment. Aching fingers aside, most doctors today cannot spare the time to use the traditional technique.

How does electroacupuncture compare to this traditional method? Not only is it quicker and more convenient for the doctor, it does not require such precise positioning of the needles and the results are far more striking. One reason for the superior results is that the electrical stimulation can be altered by the doctor to exactly suit the patient's complaint.

The needles are identical to traditional ones, but instead of being manipulated by the doctor's hand they are vibrated by a machine called an Acupunctoscope. By linking the needles to the machine, via positive and negative output leads (electrodes), a circuit is completed through which a weak electric current can pass.

The machine shown operates in the range of three to twelve volts and is best powered by an ordinary battery since this removes any danger of an electric shock, an important factor in patient relaxation!

The electric current makes the needle vibrate visibly in the skin, and the nature of the vibration can be tailor-made to suit each case. Inside the acupunctoscope is a pulse generator which can alter both the frequency (number of cycles per second) and the pulse shape of the current passing through the needle. The shape of the pulse is very important — for most treatment it will be saw-tooth, but other shapes like rectangular and sine wave are also used. Other components in the machine alter the current intensity and the duration of each pulse, which is usually in the region of two to six microseconds.

MODEL WQ-100 MULTI-PURPOSE ELECTRONIC ACUPUNCTOSCOPE.

The WQ-100 series acupunctoscope is by now the most popular acupuncture stimulator used by acupuncturist. With more than 10 years' production experience and product modification, a latest model WQ-100 has finally come out into the market which will replace all the other WQ-10's in the long run. Today, the WQ-100 is a newly designed acupunctoscope, both in its appearance, circuit, accessories, and distinguished features. It is the most powerful multi-purpose acupuncture stimulator as well as a T.E.N.S. unit.

Model IC - 1107 Electro-Acupunctoscope is also recommended

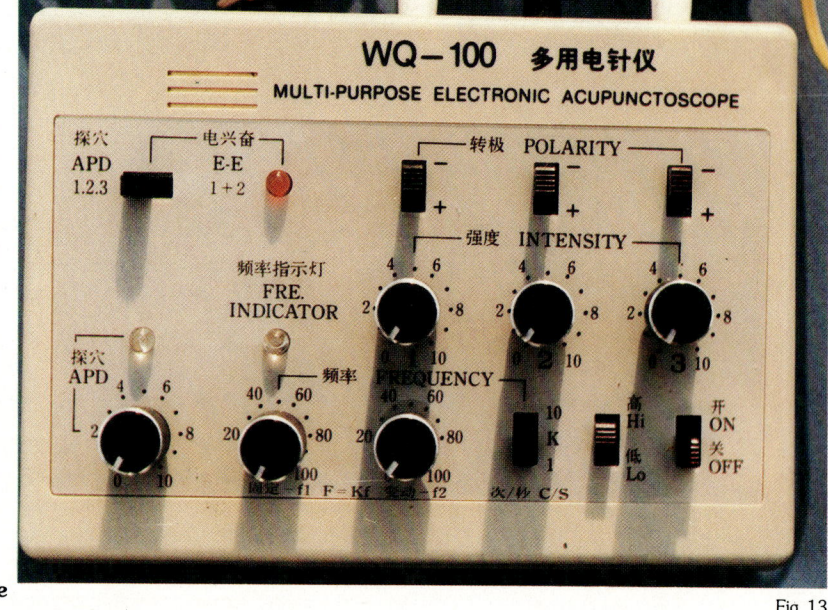

Fig. 12

Fig. 13

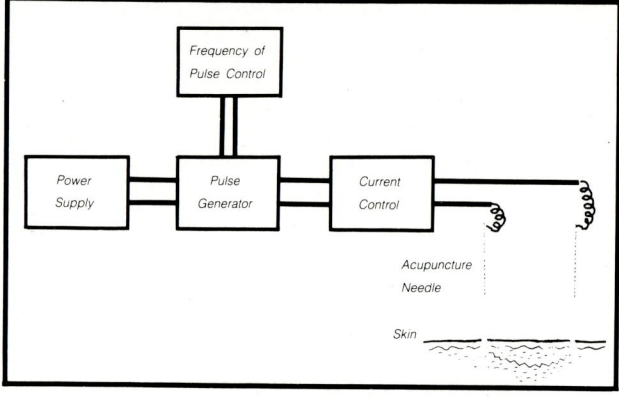

Principles of an Acupuncture Stimulator.

Advantages of Electronic Acupuncture

(1) Electronic stimulation shortens the time of treatment 5 to 10 minutes stimulated, is often the equivalent of 20 to 30 minutes unstimulated.
(2) It often reduces the number of treatments necessary.
(3) It gives a clearly-defined sedation (draining) or tonification (stimulation) effect.

Fig. 14

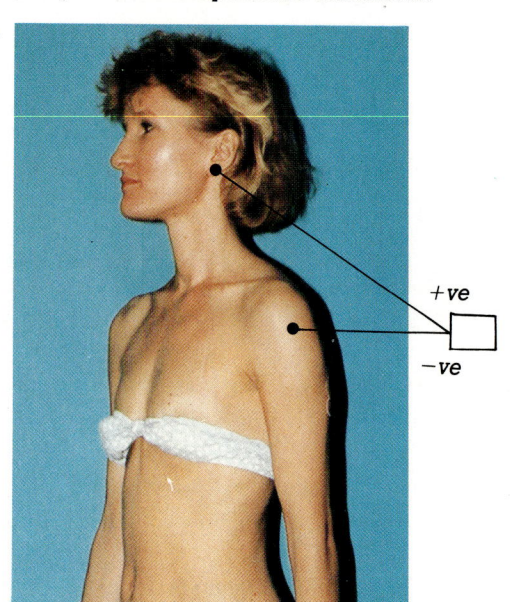

Fig. 15

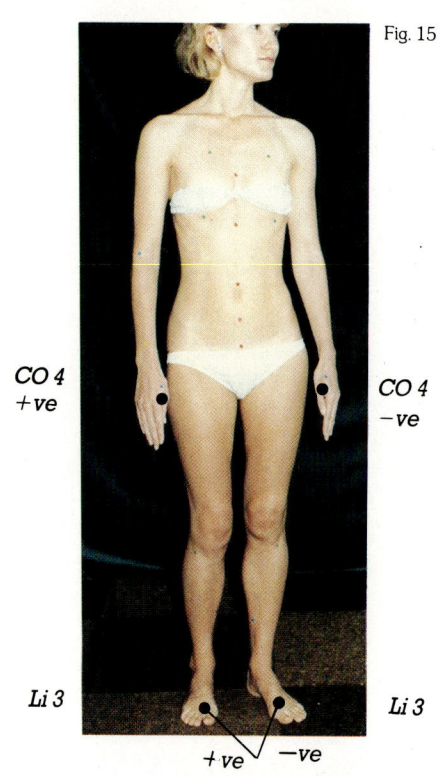

ELECTRO-ACUPUNCTURE

The Connection of Electrodes

The following points must be adhered to when connecting Electrodes to needles in patient from Electro-Acupunctoscope.

A. All positive electrodes (red) must be connected to one side of the body and all negative (black) to the other side.

B. In Auricular Therapy never ever connect positive (red) and negative (black) terminals from the same output to one ear.

C. If only one ear point is used the other terminal is connected to a body point.

D. Never ever use Electro-Acupuncture in a patient who has a pace-maker.

E. It is acceptable to connect the positive lead to a point in the right ear, and the negative lead to a different Acupuncture point in the left ear.

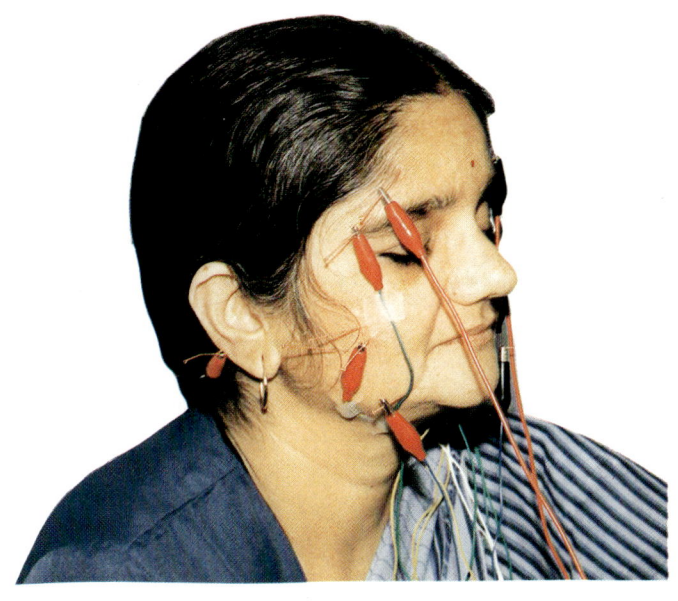

Fig. 16

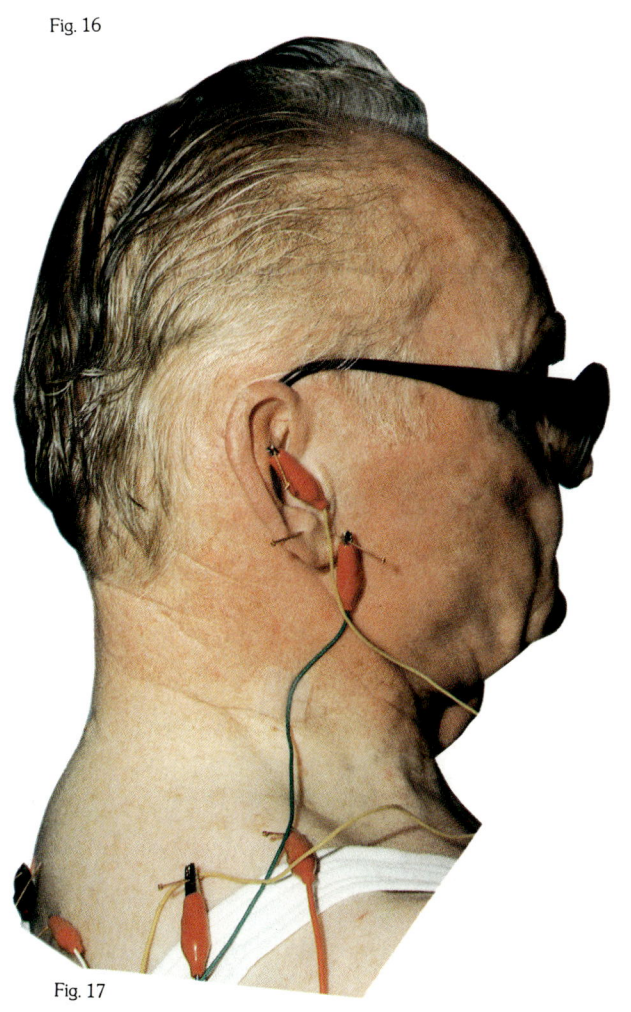

Fig. 17

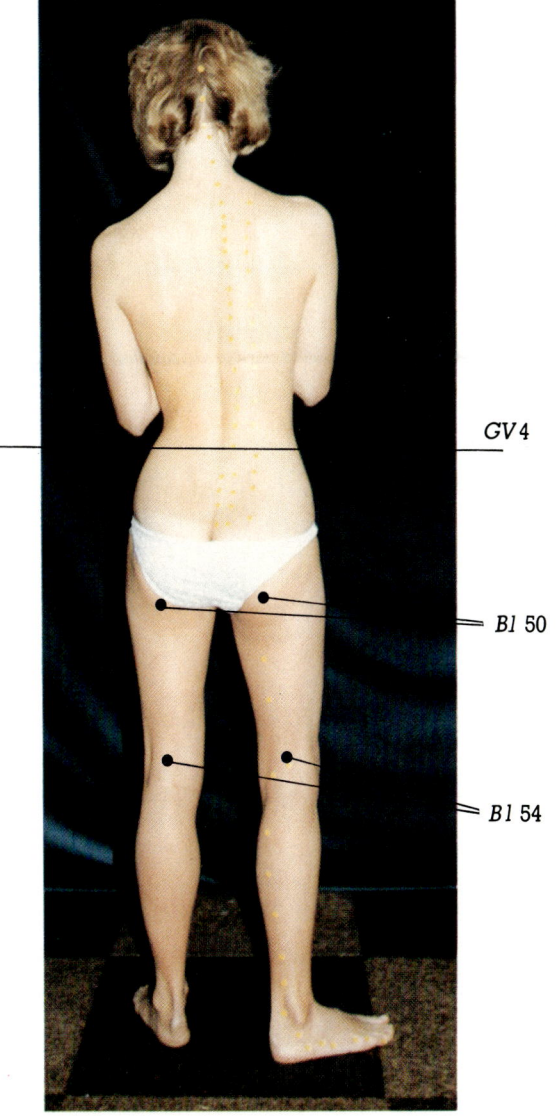

GV 4

Bl 50

Bl 54

17

The 12 Ordinary Meridians and the two Extra Ordinary Meridians

The Ordinary Meridians:—

1. Twelve pairs.
2. Bilateral — represented on both sides of the body, e.g.

   Colon 1 (CO.1) is on the radial side of the index finger — right and left of the index finger and the nail points.

   Pericardium 6 (P.6) is represented in both forearms on the flexor surface 2" above the wrist crease.

   Spleen 6 (Sp.6) is 3" above the medial malleolus in a depression in both legs on the medial aspect. This point is important as 3 Meridians meet at this point. (Sp.6, K.7, L.6)

The Extra-ordinary Meridians:—

1. Two in number.
2. They are single.
3. The Governor Meridian is in the dorsal surface in the midline — 28 points.
4. The Conception Vessel is in the ventral surface in the midline — 24 points.

Meridians:— Clinically there is abundant evidence to indicate the existence of reflex links between Acupuncture points and specific organs and their functions.

CUN = AUM = Acupuncture Unit of Measurement.
It is the "Human Inch", the AUM of the Forearm Ex. is determined by measuring the distance between the wrist crease and the cubital crease and dividing it by 12. The Human Inch - The CUN varies with patient to patient.

Always refer to section 3 - Body Acupuncture Meridians and Section 11 - Ear Acupuncture, Cartography and Ear points if you are not sure of a location of a certain point - when referring to other sections of the Atlas or in treating a patient.

Yang +VE Meridians shown in Red

Yin −VE Meridians shown in Black

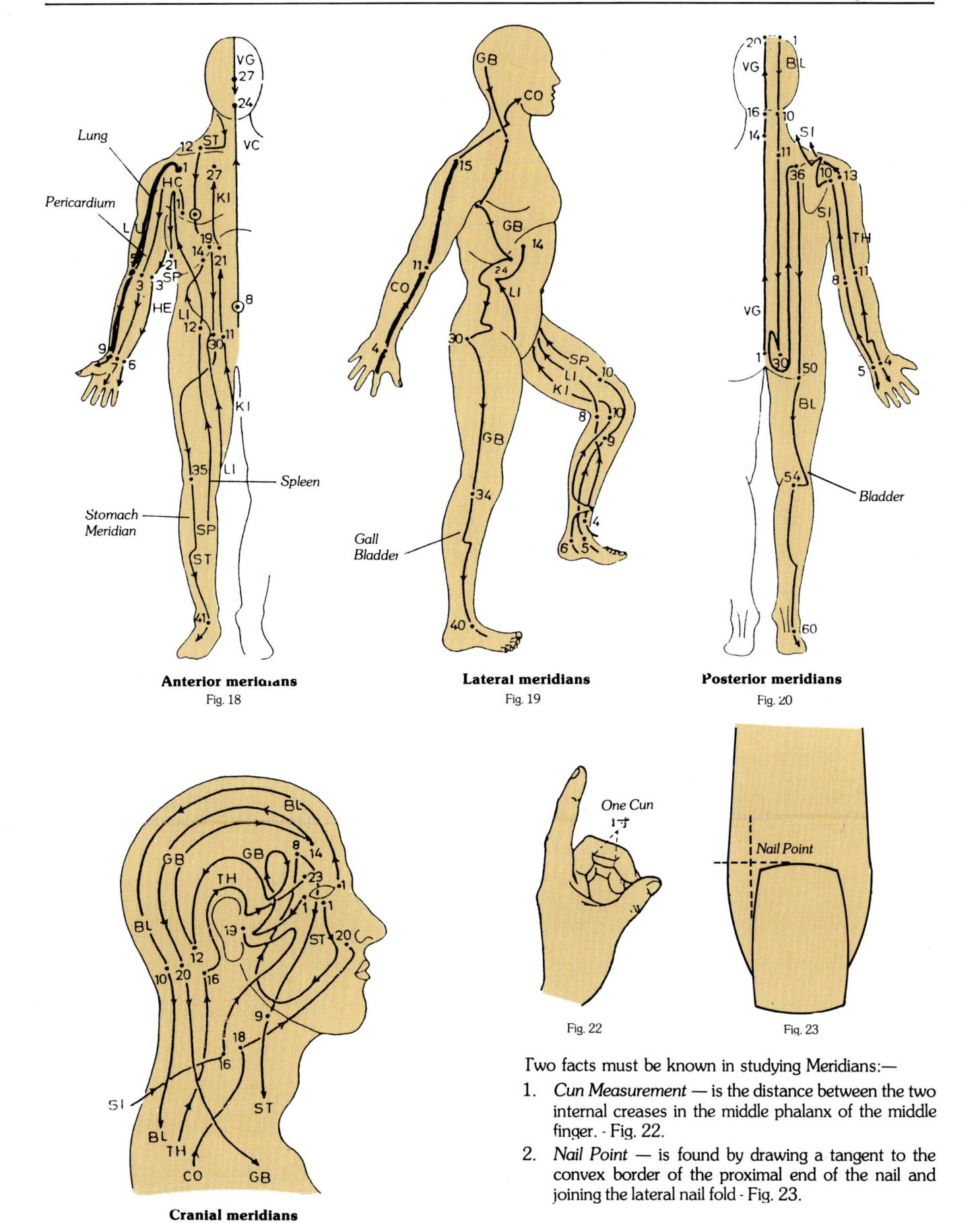

THE 12 ORDINARY MERIDIANS

Anterior meridians
Fig. 18

Lateral meridians
Fig. 19

Posterior meridians
Fig. 20

Cranial meridians
Fig. 21

Fig. 22

Fig. 23

Two facts must be known in studying Meridians:—

1. *Cun Measurement* — is the distance between the two internal creases in the middle phalanx of the middle finger. - Fig. 22.
2. *Nail Point* — is found by drawing a tangent to the convex border of the proximal end of the nail and joining the lateral nail fold - Fig. 23.

THE 12 ORDINARY MERIDIANS

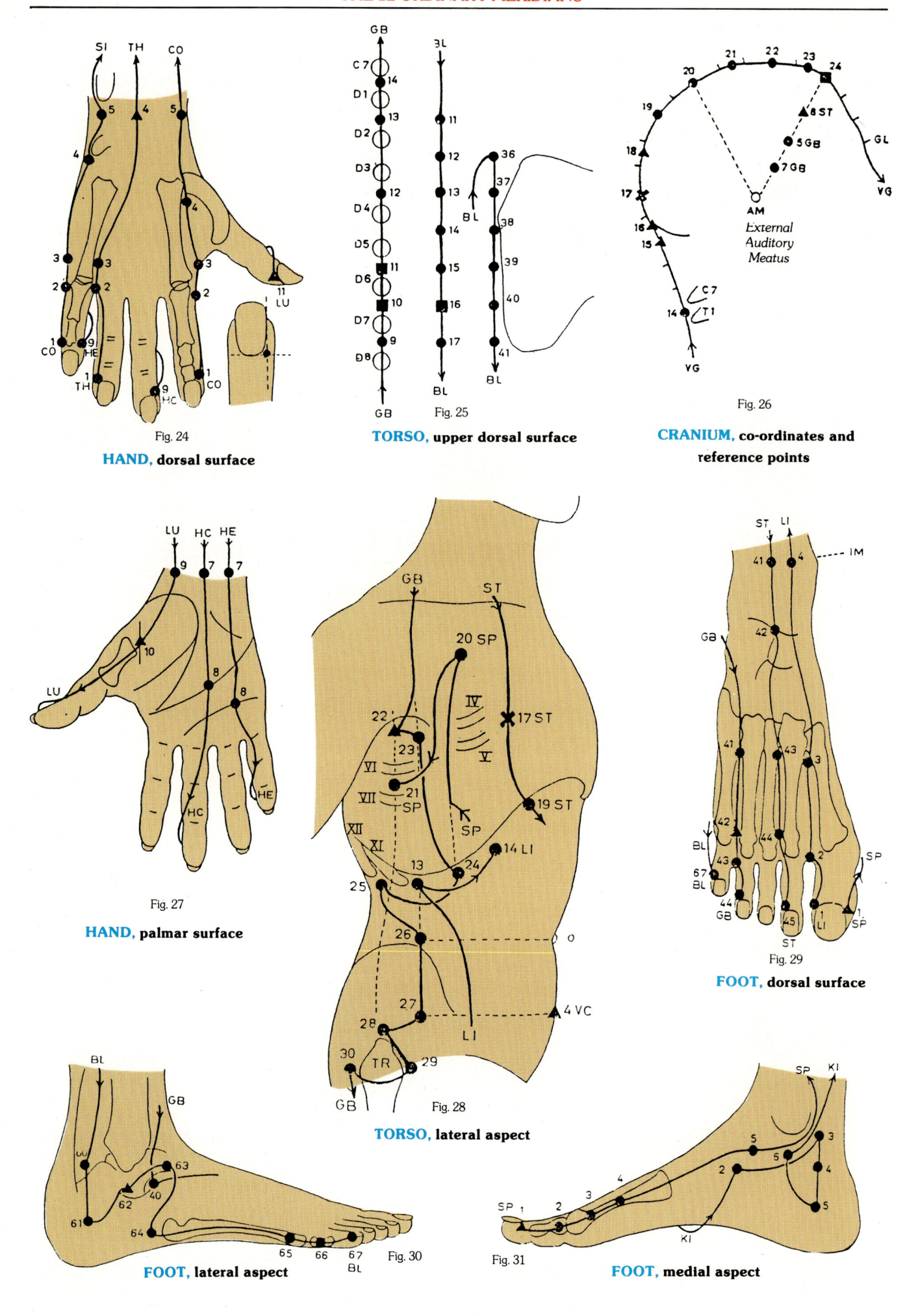

Fig. 24
HAND, dorsal surface

Fig. 25
TORSO, upper dorsal surface

Fig. 26
CRANIUM, co-ordinates and reference points

Fig. 27
HAND, palmar surface

Fig. 28
TORSO, lateral aspect

Fig. 29
FOOT, dorsal surface

Fig. 30
FOOT, lateral aspect

Fig. 31
FOOT, medial aspect

THE 12 ORDINARY MERIDIANS

Fig. 32

Lu 2
Lu 1
Lu 3
Lu 4
Lu 5
Lu 6
Lu 7
Lu 8
Lu 9
Lu 10
Lu 11

Lung Meridian

Fig. 33

Co. 19
Co. 20
Co. 15
Co. 18
Co. 17
Co. 14
Co. 13
Co. 12
Co. 11
Co. 10
Co. 9
Co. 8
Co. 7
Co. 6
Co. 5
Co. 4
Co. 3
Co. 2
Co. 1

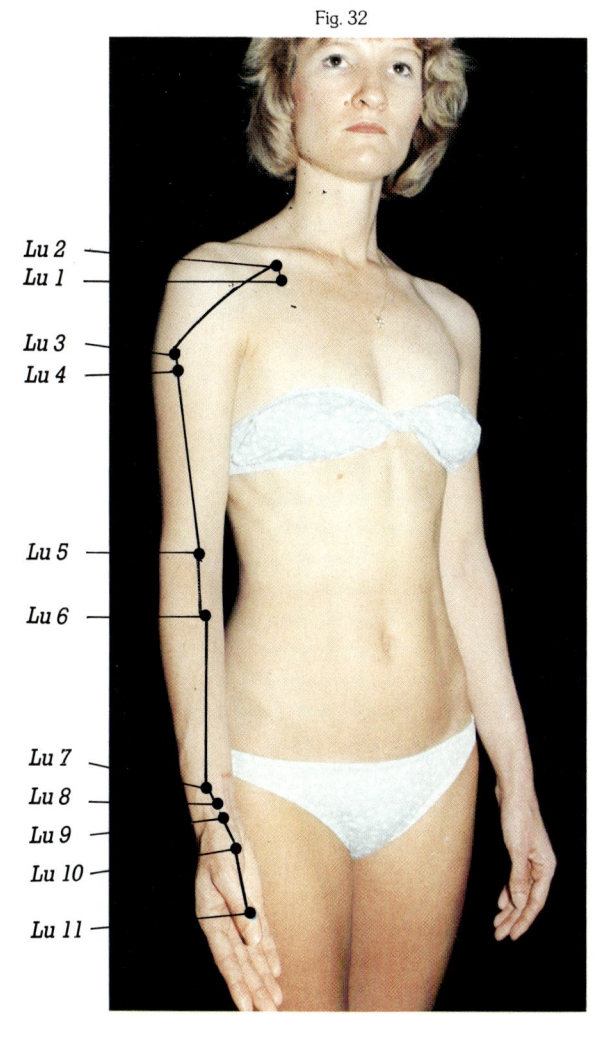

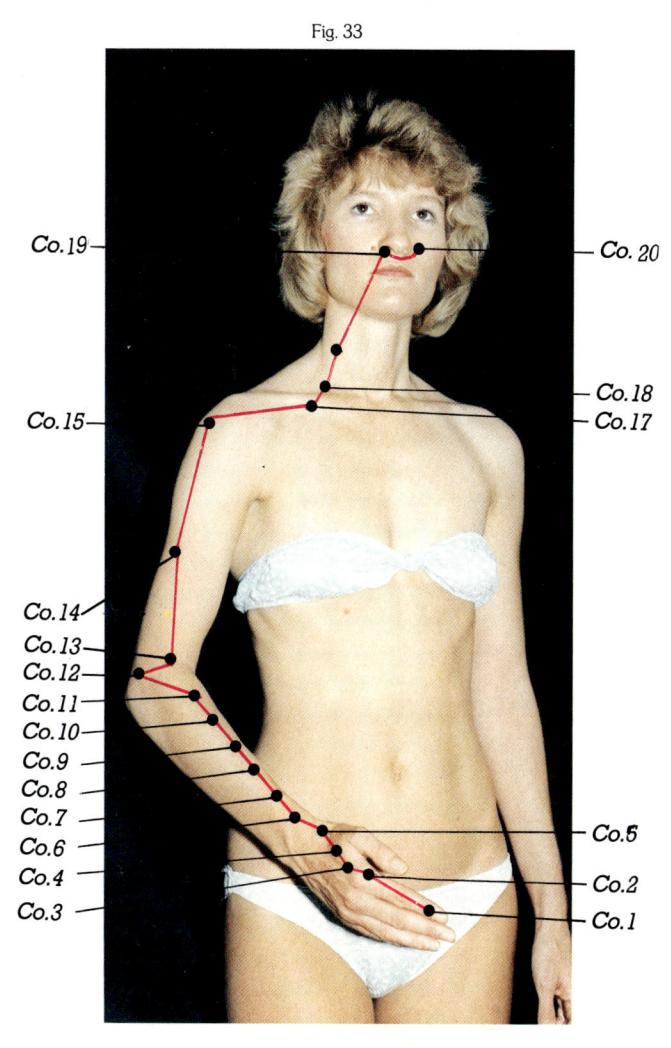

Colon Meridian

LUNG MERIDIAN

LUNG MERIDIAN has 11 Acupuncture Points.
Important points of the Meridian are:—

LU.1.   6" from midline, 2nd inter-space.

LU.2.   Tip of coracoid process.

LU.5.   Lateral to the bicipital tendon when elbow is flexed.

LU.7.   Superior to the styloid process of the radius 1.5" above the transverse crease of the wrist.

LU.9.   At the transverse crease of the wrist in a depression on the radial side.

LU.11. At the nail point.

COLON MERIDIAN

COLON MERIDIAN has 20 Acupuncture Points.
Important Points are:—

CO.1.   Nail Point, index finger on the radial side.

CO.4.   Is the most important point. Between the 1st and 2nd metacarpals.

CO.11. In the region of the elbow at the lateral end of the crease when the elbow is flexed.

CO.15. At the depression of the shoulder when the arm is fully abducted.

CO.19. Directly below the lateral margin of the nostril.

CO.20. In the nasalobial groove at the level of the midpoint of ala nasi.

THE 12 ORDINARY MERIDIANS

Fig. 34

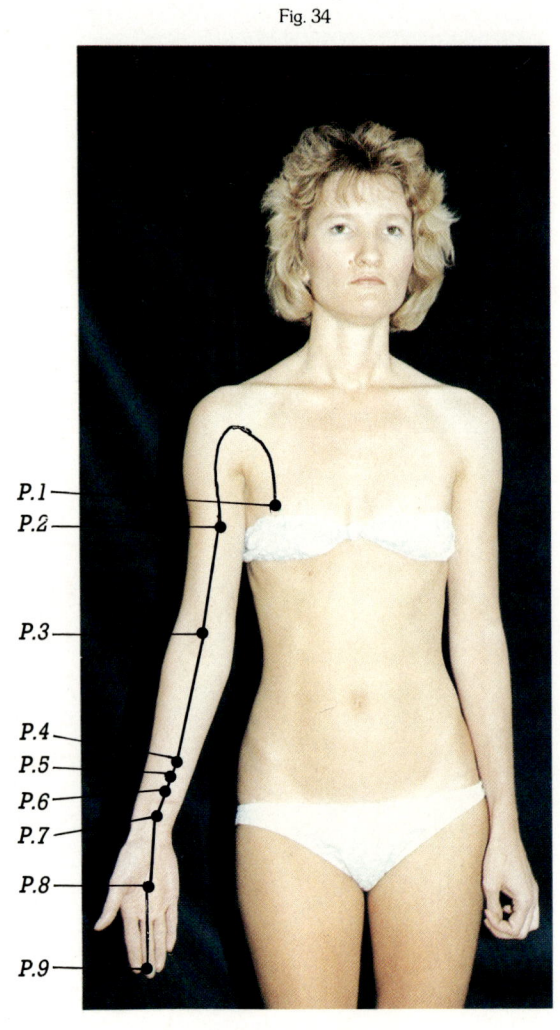

Fig. 35

Pericardium Meridian

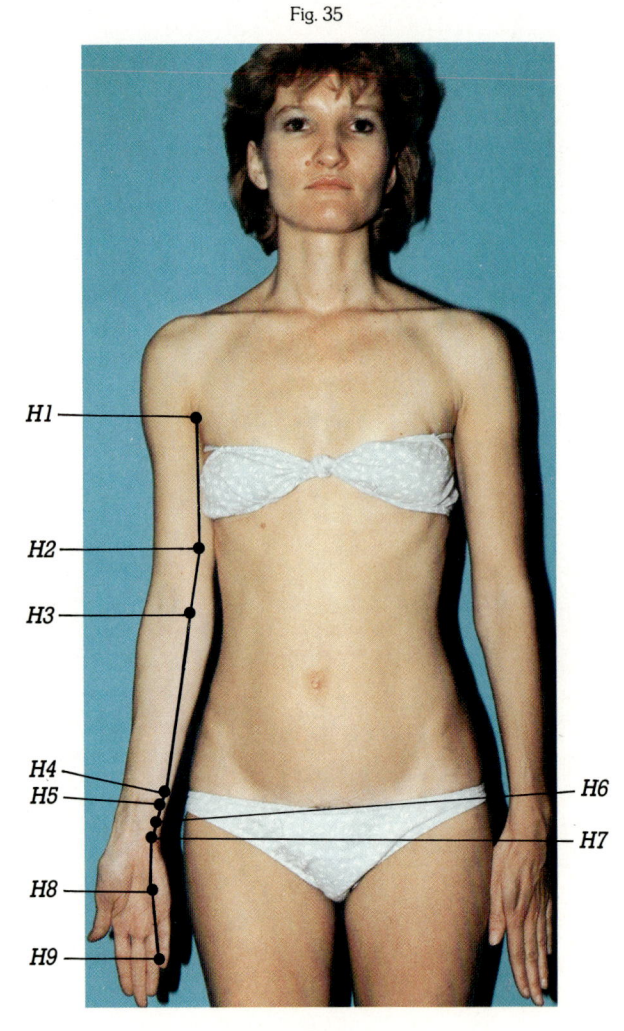

Heart Meridian

PERICARDIUM MERIDIAN

PERICARDIUM is a Yin Meridian with 9 Acupuncture Points.

Important Points of the Meridian are:—

P.1. 1″ lateral to the nipple in the 4th intercostal space.

P.3. On the transverse cubital crease at the ulna side of tendon of biceps.

P.6. 2″ above the transverse crease of the wrist.

P.7. Middle of the transverse crease of the wrist.

P.8. In the centre of the tip of the middle finger

HEART MERIDIAN

HEART MERIDIAN is a Yin Meridian with 9 Acupuncture Points.

the Important Points are:-

H.1. In the centre of the axilla.

H.4. On the radial side of the tendon of the flexor carpi ulnaris muscle 1½″ above the transverse crease of the wrist.

H.7. On the transverse crease of the wrist between the pisiform bone and the ulna.

H.9. Nail Point on the lateral aspect of the little finger.

THE 12 ORDINARY MERIDIANS

Fig. 36

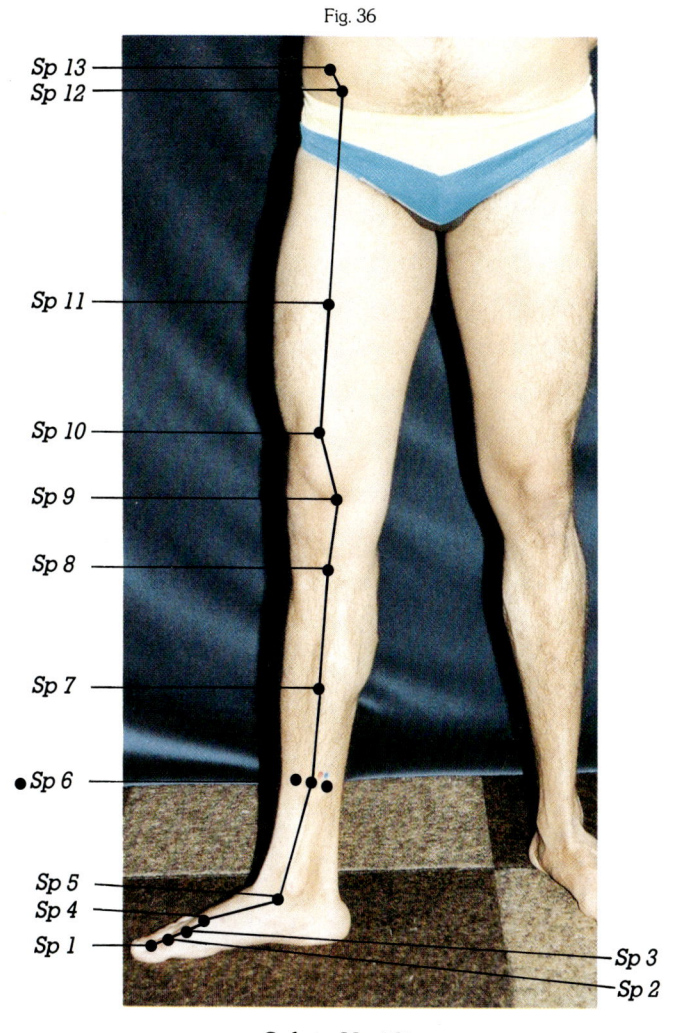

Fig. 37

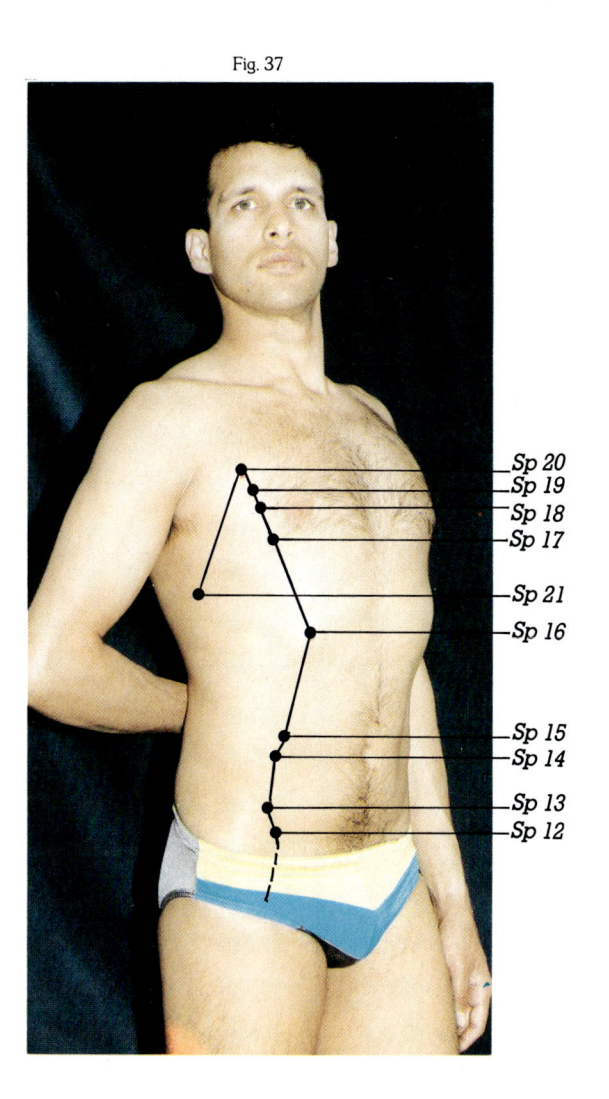

Spleen Meridian

SPLEEN MERIDIAN

SPLEEN MERIDIAN is a Yin Meridian, component of the earth element with 21 Acupuncture Points.

Important Points of the Meridian are:—

Sp. 1   Nail point medial side of the big toe.

Sp. 6   It is a very important point 3 inches above the medial malleolus. Three Meridians — Spleen, Liver and Kidney — cross here. Used in Gynaecology problems, Nervous Tension, etc. Acupuncture of Sp. 6 is contra indicated during pregnancy.

Sp. 10 2" above and medial to the patella.

Sp. 11 6" above Sp. 10 on the line drawn from Sp. 10 to Sp. 12.

Sp. 15 4" lateral to the centre of the umbilicus on the mammillary line.

Sp. 16 3" above Sp. 15.

Sp. 18 2" lateral to the nipple in the 4th Intercostal space.

Sp. 21 Mid-axillary line 6" below the axilla (6th intercostal space), lateral to rectus abdominis muscle.

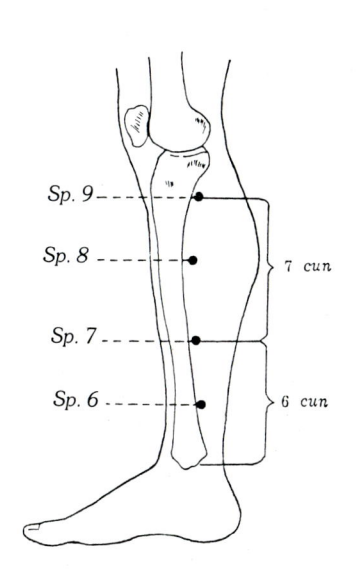

25

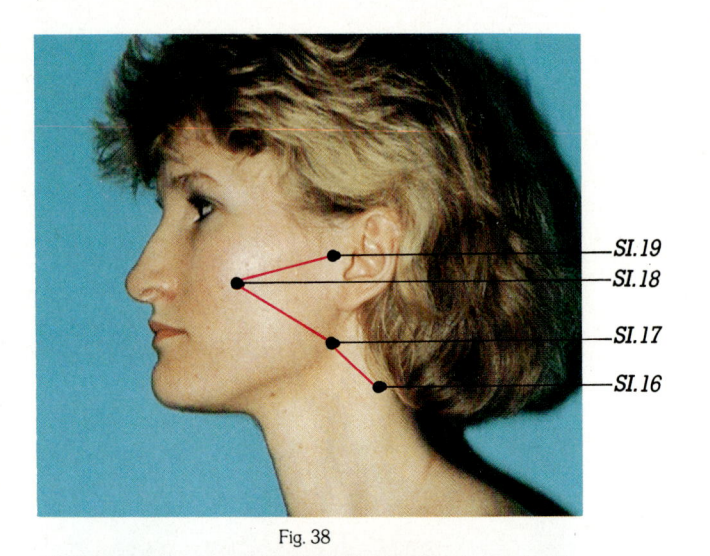

THE 12 ORDINARY MERIDIANS

SMALL INTESTINE MERIDIAN

SMALL INTESTINE is a Yang component of the fire element with 19 Acupuncture Points.

Important points of the Meridian are:—

S.I.1	On the medial side of the little finger, Nail Point.
S.I.3	At the end of the heart line on the medial aspect of the palm.
S.I.6	Dorsal to the head of the ulna.
S.I.8	Between the olecranon of the ulna and the medial epicondyle.
S.I.12	In the centre of the scapular directly above S.I.11.
S.I.18	Directly below the outer canthus in the depression on the lower border of zygoma.
S.I.19	Between the tragus and the mandibular joint.

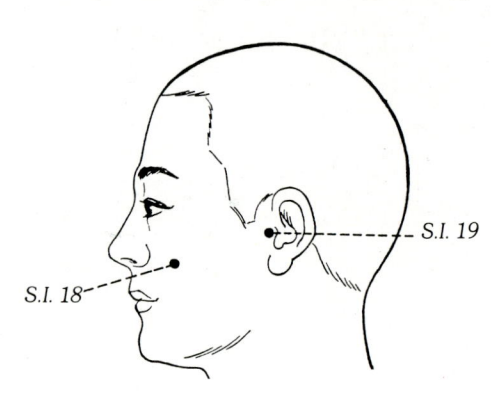

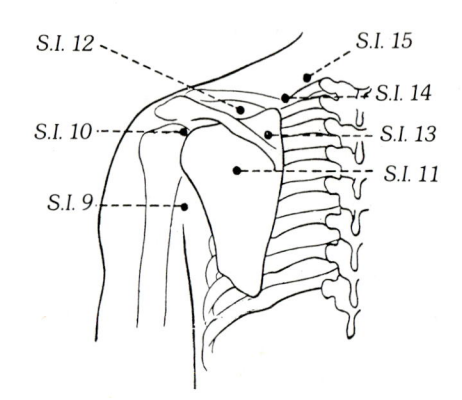

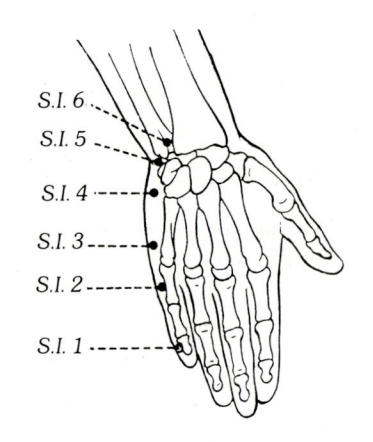

Fig. 38

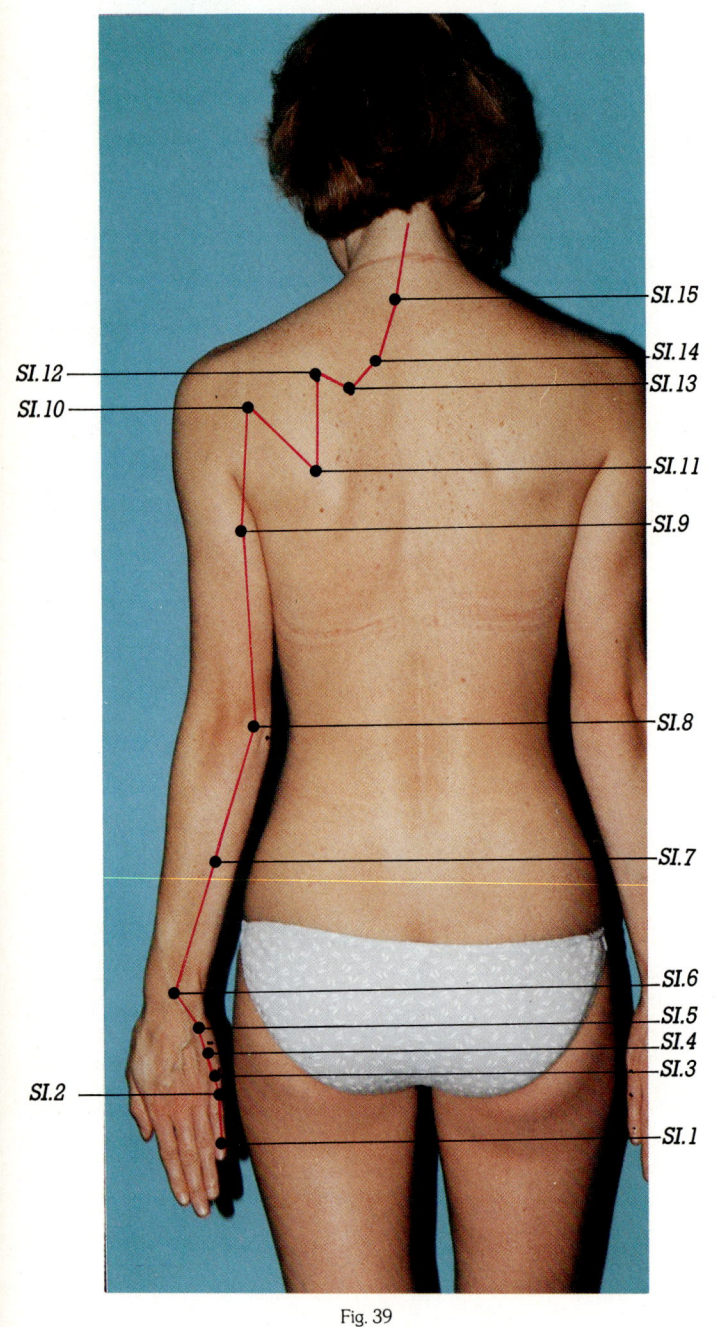

Fig. 39

Small Intestine Meridian

26

THE 12 ORDINARY MERIDIANS

Fig. 40

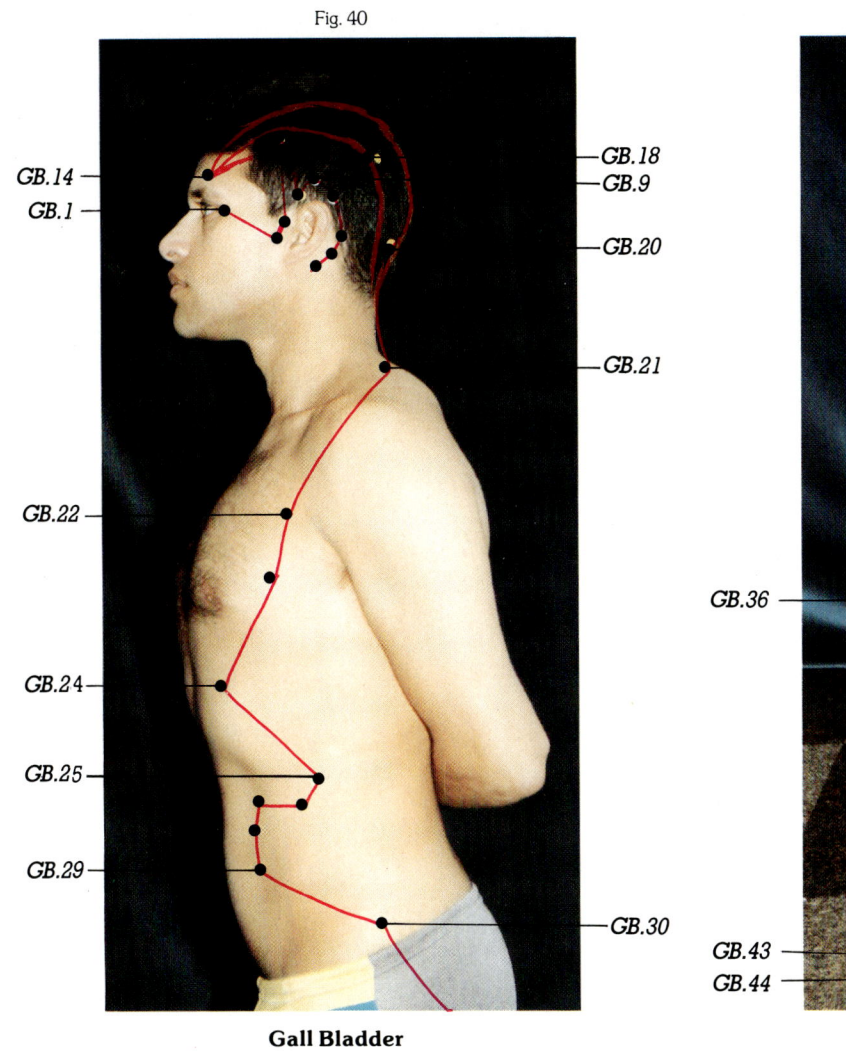

Gall Bladder

Fig. 41

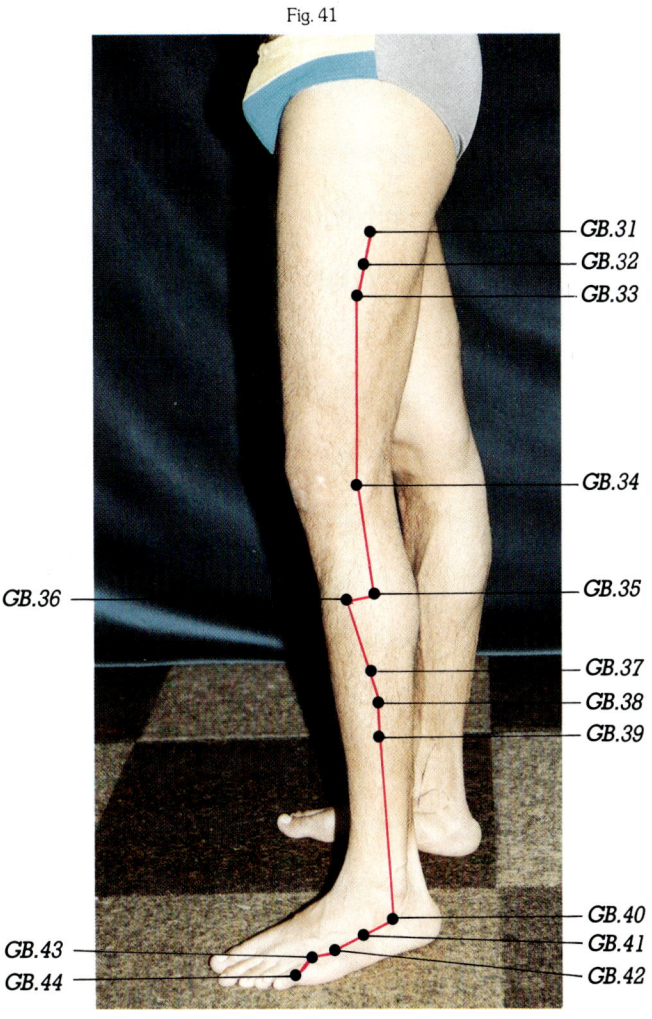

Gall Bladder

GALL BLADDER

GALL BLADDER is a Yang Meridian of the wood element with 44 Acupuncture Points.

Important Points are:—

GB.1   Lateral to the outer canthus below TH.23.

GB.2   Anterior to the intertragic notch, directly below S.I. 19.

GB.14 On the forehead 1″ above the midpoint of the eyebrow.

GB.20 In the posterior aspect of the neck in the depression between the upper portion of sterno-mastoideus and trapezius.

GB.21 In the middle of supraclavicular fossa, midway between GV. 14 and the acromion - Fig. 39a

GB.34 In the depression anterior and inferior to the head of the fibula.

GB.35 7″ above the tip of the lateral malleolus, on the posterior border of the fibula.

GB.36 7″ above the tip of the lateral malleolus on the anterior border of the fibula.

GB.37 5″ directly above the tip of the lateral malleolus.

GB.41 In the depression distal to the conjunction of the 4th and 5th metatarsal bone.

GB.44 On the lateral side of the 4th toe-nail point.

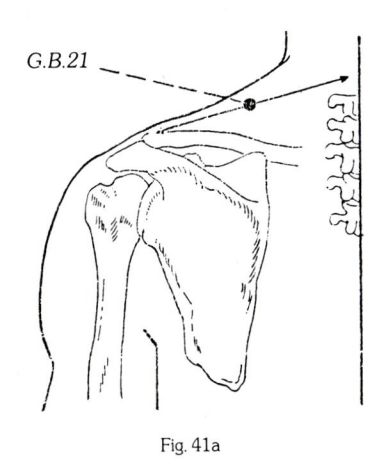

Fig. 41a

THE 12 ORDINARY MERIDIANS

Fig. 42

UB 10
UB 11
UB 12
UB 17
UB 18
UB 21
UB 23
UB 31
UB 32
UB 33
UB 34
UB 36
UB 40
UB 27
UB 48
UB 49
UB 30

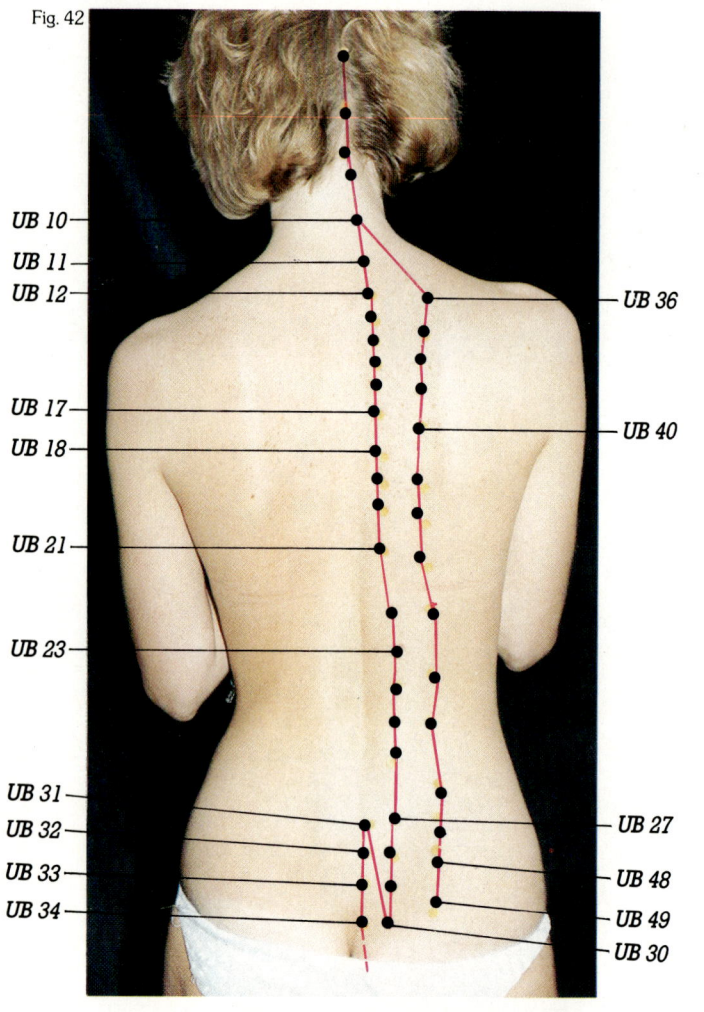

Bladder Meridian

Fig. 43

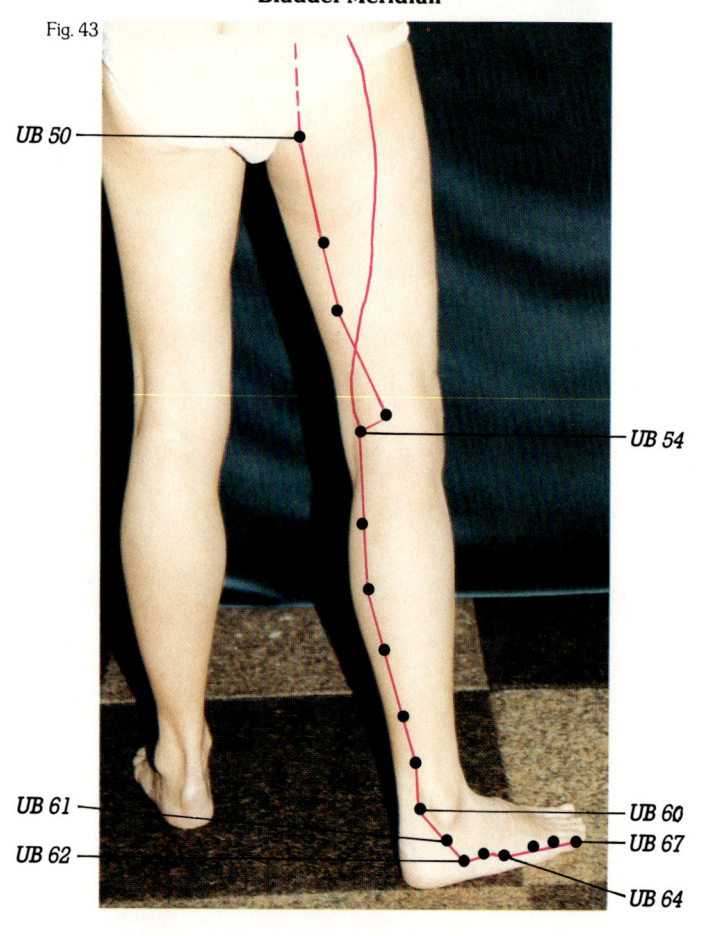

UB 50
UB 54
UB 61
UB 62
UB 60
UB 67
UB 64

Fig. 44

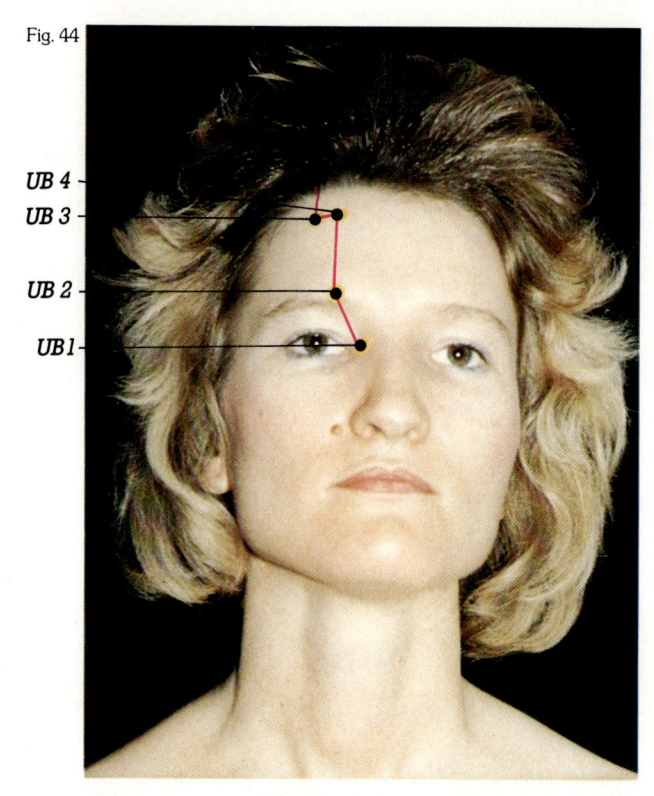

UB 4
UB 3
UB 2
UB 1

Bladder Meridian

BLADDER MERIDIAN

BLADDER is a Yang Meridian, Yang component of the water element with 67 Acupuncture Points.

Important Points of the Meridian are:—

B.1	0.1″ superior to the inner canthus
B.2	On the supraorbital notch.
B.3	Directly above the medial extremity of the eyebrow 1 cun above B.2.
B.8	1½″ posterior to B.7, 1½″ lateral to the Governor Meridian.
B.10	1½″ lateral to G.15 within posterior hairline.
B.11	From midline 1½″ lateral to the Governor Meridian.
B.11/30	All in the same line drawn 1½″ from midline in the line joining B.11 to B.30 which is at level of the 4th posterior sacral foramen.
B.31/34	Are in the corresponding posterior sacral foramen 1 to 4.
B.36	At the level of B.12, 3″ from midline. 36 to 49 are in the plum line dropped from the medial border in the body of the scapula.
B.50	In the middle of the gluteal fold.
B.54	In the middle of the popliteal crease.
B.60	Just posterior to the lateral malleolus.
B.64	In the styloid process of the 5th metatarsal.
B.67	Nail point specific for labour and gynaecological problems.

THE 12 ORDINARY MERIDIANS

Fig. 45

Ki 27
Ki 22
Ki 21
Ki 15
Umbilicus
Ki 11
Ki 10
Ki 9
Ki 8
Ki 3
Ki 6
Ki 2
Ki 4
Ki 5

Kidney Meridian

Fig. 46

Li 14
Li 13
Li 12
Li 10
Li 8
Li 5
Li 3
Li 1

Liver Meridian

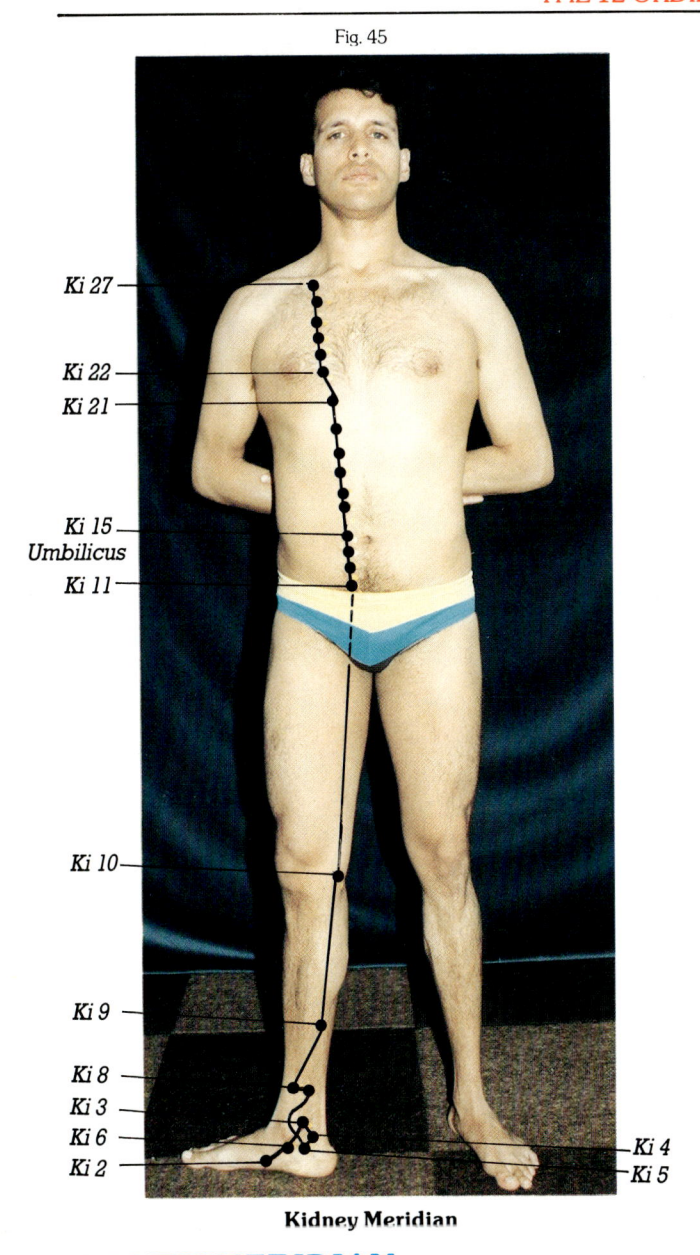

KIDNEY MERIDIAN

KIDNEY MERIDIAN is a Yin Meridian with 27 Acupuncture Points.

Important Points of the Meridian are:—

K.1 In the depression of the sole when the foot is in plantar flexion approximately at the junction of the anterior third and posterior two-thirds.

K.2 Anterior and inferior to the medial malleolus.

K.6 1 cun below the medial malleolus.

K.7 2″ above the medial malleolus in the region of Spleen 6.

K.11 5″ below the umbilicus on the superior border of the symphysis pubis ½″ lateral to the midline.

K.21 6″ above umbilicus ½″ lateral to the midline and to Conception point 14.

K.22 In the 5th intercostal space 2″ lateral to the midline.

K.27 In the depression on the lower border of the clavicle 2″ lateral to midline.

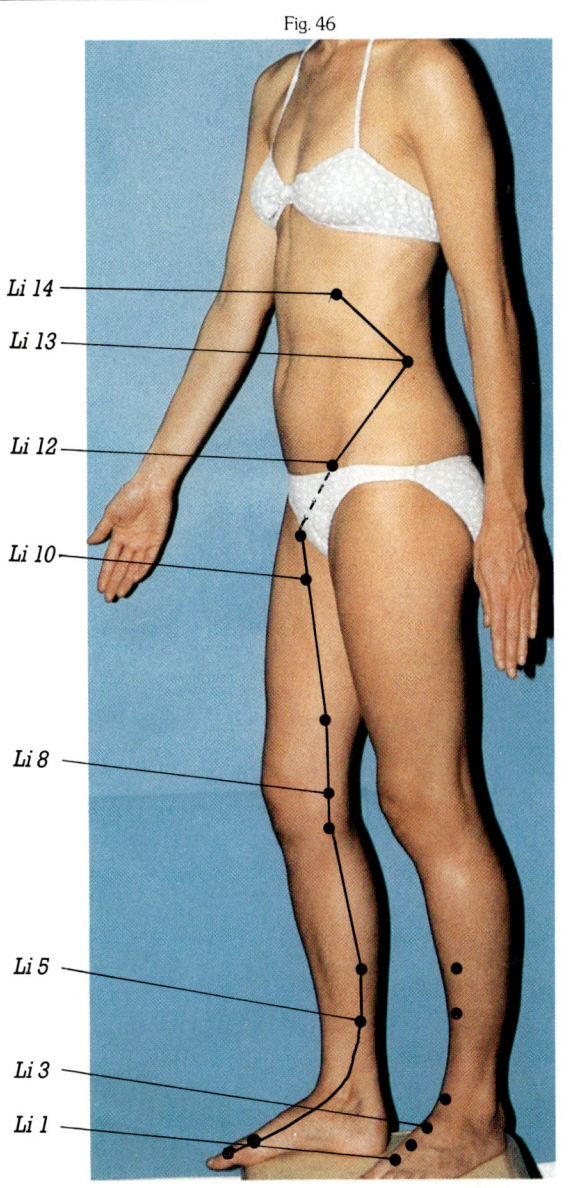

LIVER MERIDIAN

LIVER MERIDIAN IS A Yin Meridian with 14 Acupuncture Points.

Important points of the Meridian are:—

L.1 Nail point lateral side of big toe.

L.3 Between the 1st and 2nd metatarsal bones.

L.7 Posterior and inferior to the medial condyle of the tibia.

L.13 On the lateral side of the abdomen below the free end of the 11th floating rib.

L.14 On the mammillary line in the 6th intercostal space.

THE 12 ORDINARY MERIDIANS

THREE HEATER MERIDIAN

THREE HEATER is a Yang Meridian with 23 Acupuncture Points.

Important Points are:—

TH.1   Lateral side of the ring finger at nail point.

TH.5   3″ above the wrist crease between the radius and ulna.

TH.10   When the elbow is flexed, the point is in the depression about 1″ superior to the olecranon.

TH.16   Is posterior and inferior to the mastoid process. It is a nervous tension point. (N.T.)

TH.23   In the depression at the lateral end of the eyebrow.

Fig. 47 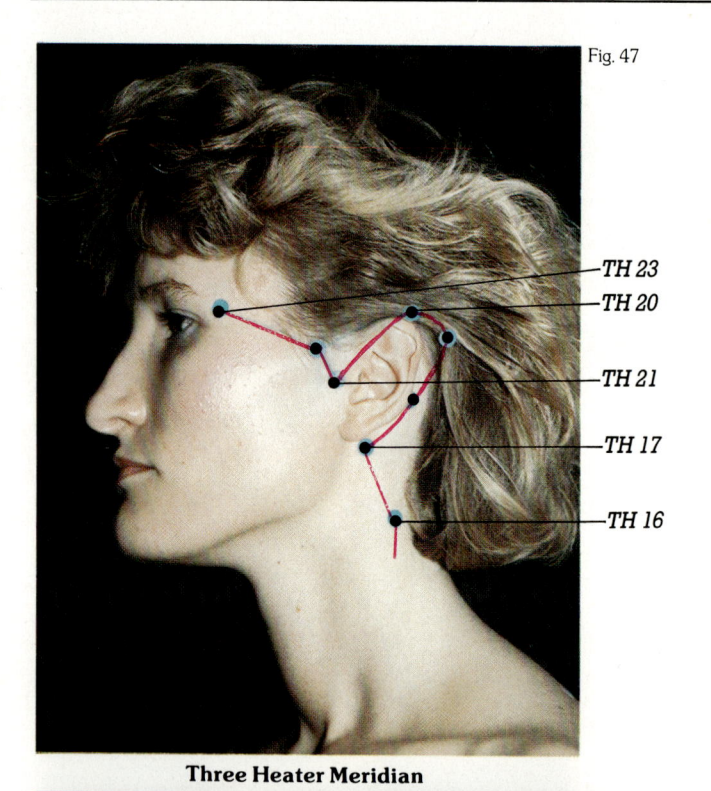
Three Heater Meridian

Fig. 48 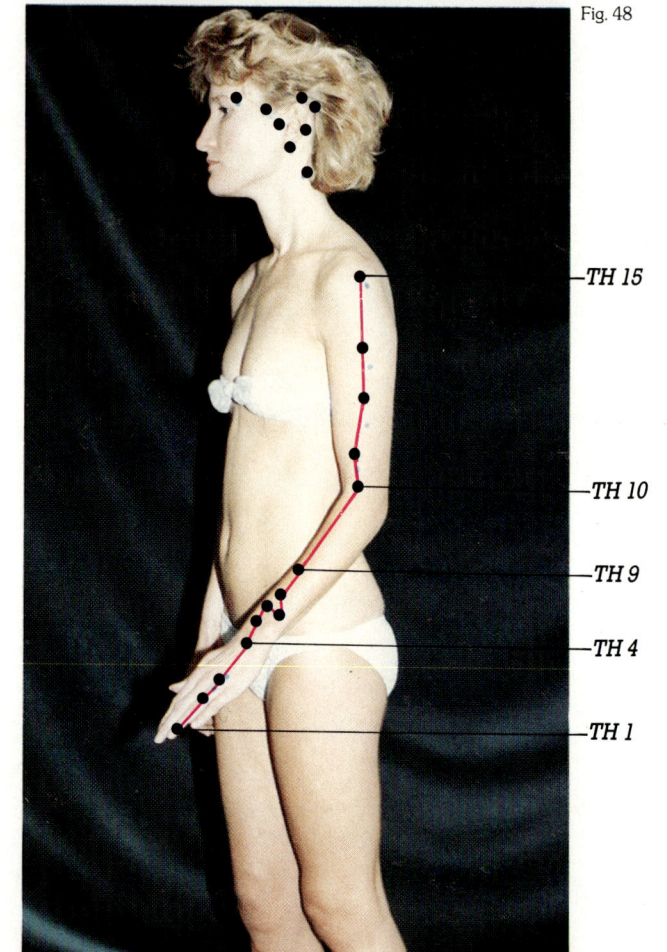
Three Heater Meridian

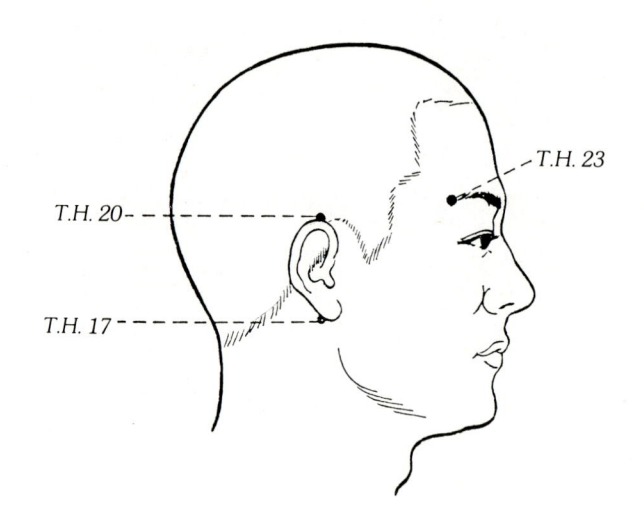

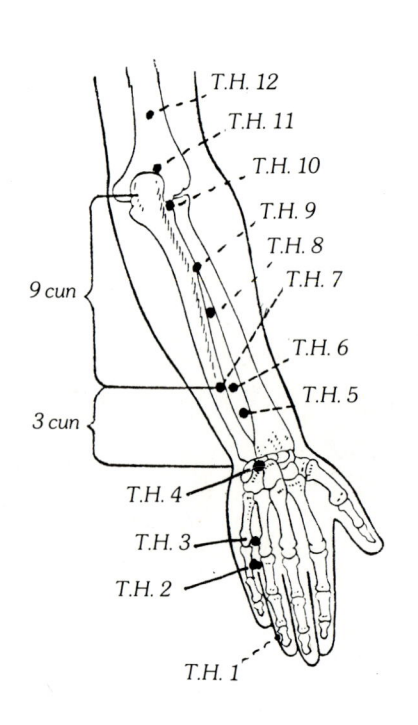

THE 12 ORDINARY MERIDIANS

Fig. 49

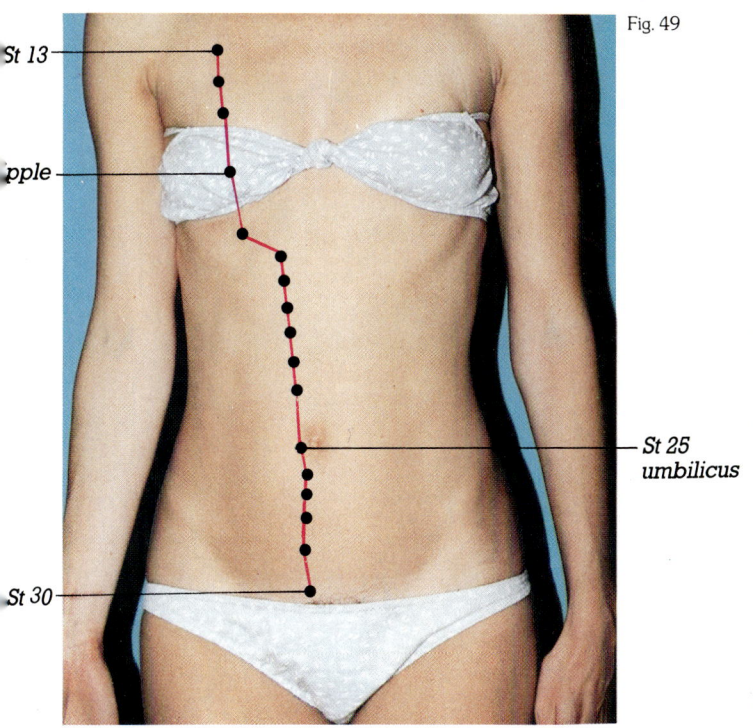

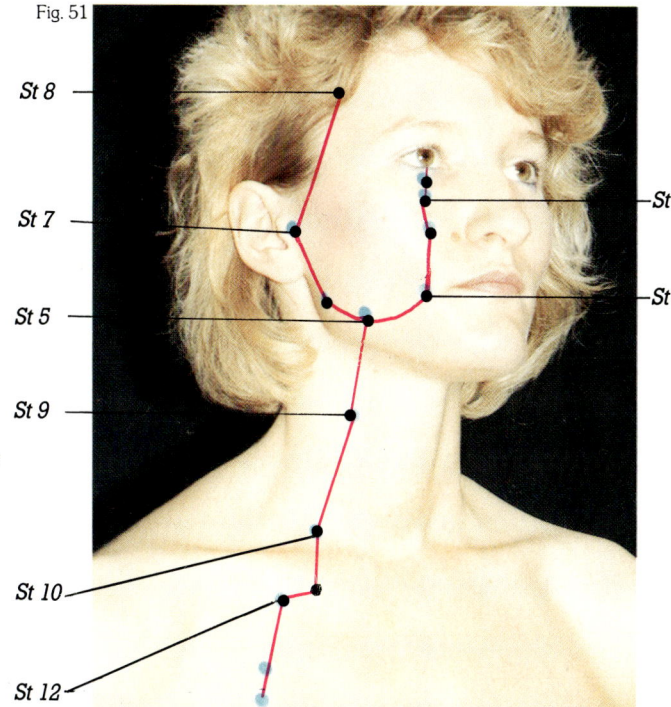

St 13
pple
St 25 umbilicus
St 30

Stomach Meridian

Fig. 50

St 31
St 35
St 36
St 41
St 44
St 45 NAIL PT.

Fig. 51

St 8
St 7
St 5
St 9
St 10
St 12
St 2
St 4

Stomach Meridian

STOMACH MERIDIAN

STOMACH is a Yang component of the earth element with 45 Acupuncture Points.

Important Points of the Meridian are:—

St.1	In the lower eye lid in the line of the pupil.
St.2	Infra-orbital foramen.
St.3	In the same line lateral to the nose.
St.4	In the same line lateral to the angle of the mouth.
St.5/6	Anterior and posterior to the masseter muscle.
St.7	In front of the tragus.
St.8	Just above the hairline.
St.9	Level of the thyroid cartilage joining St.5.
St.12	Upper border middle of clavicle.
St.17	Nipple — 4th intercostal space.
St.18	1″ below St.17.
St.19	6″ above the umbilicus 2″ lateral to the midline.
St.25	2″ lateral to the centre of the umbilicus.
St.36	Anterior to the head of the fibula below the knee.
St.40	In the line of the 2nd toe between the lateral and medial malleolus.
St.43	In the depression distal to the junction of the 2nd and 3rd metatarsal bones.
St.45	Nail point 2nd toe lateral side.

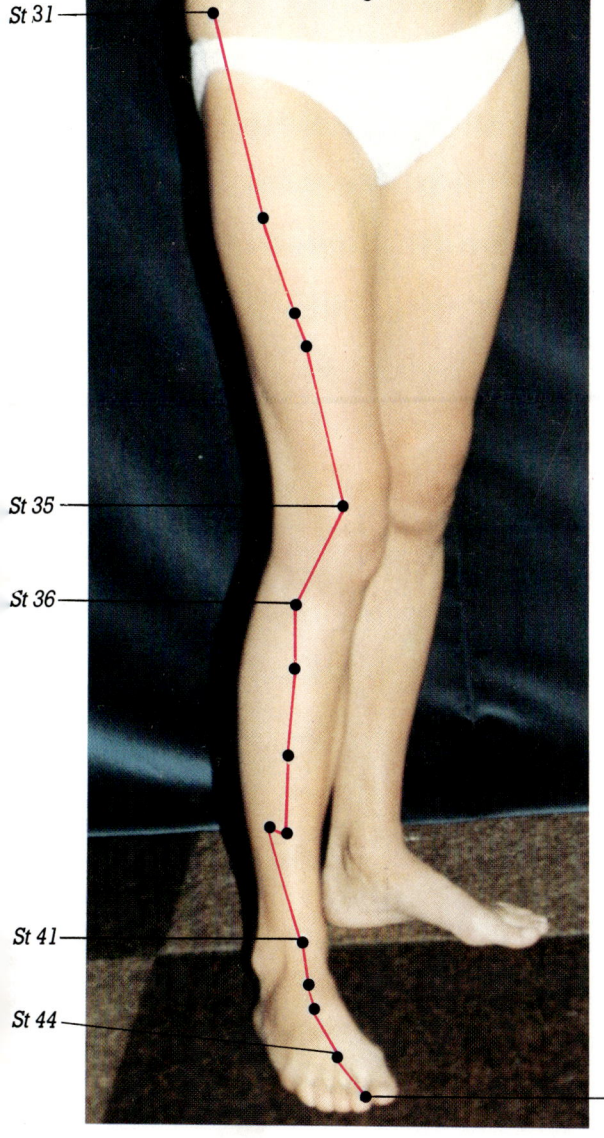

The Extra-Ordinary Meridians

1. Ren or Conception Meridian
2. Governor or Du Meridian
3. Nail points in the Foot and the Hand
4. Meeran's Laws for Meridians
5. Nail Point
6. Cun Measurement

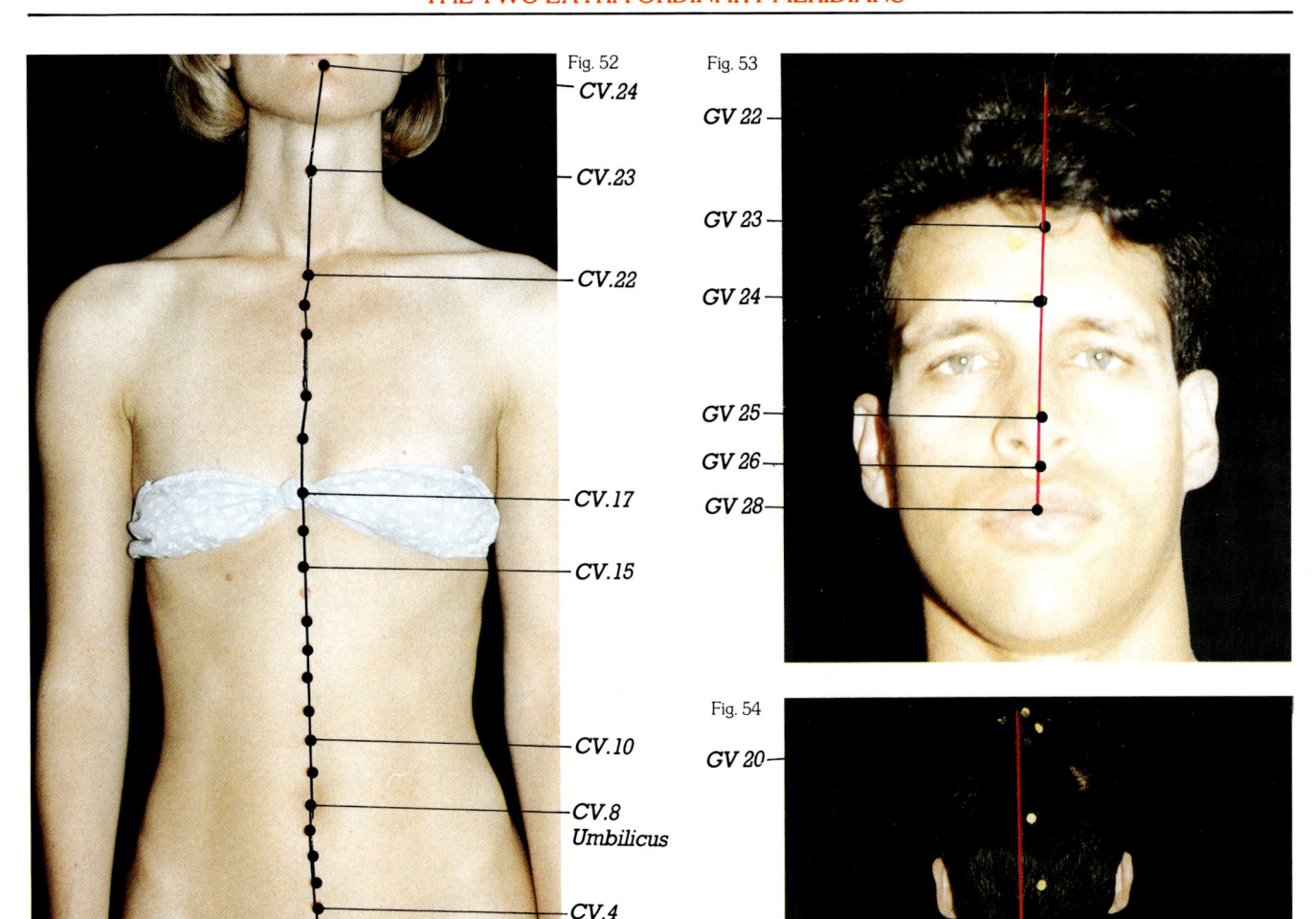

THE TWO EXTRA ORDINARY MERIDIANS

Fig. 52
- CV.24
- CV.23
- CV.22
- CV.17
- CV.15
- CV.10
- CV.8 Umbilicus
- CV.4
- CV.2

Fig. 53
- GV 22
- GV 23
- GV 24
- GV 25
- GV 26
- GV 28

Fig. 54
- GV 20
- GV 14(C7)
- GV 12(T6)
- GV 6(T12)
- GV 4(L2)
- GV 2

REN OR CONCEPTION MERIDIAN

REN or CONCEPTION MERIDIAN is an extra-ordinary meridian, single on the ventral surface of the midline, with 24 Acupuncture Points.

Important points of the Meridian are:—

CV.1	In the centre of the perineum.
CV.2	Midline — above symphysis pubis.
CV.8	In the centre umbilicus.
CV.15	Below the xyphoid process.
CV.23	In the notch of the thyroid cartilage.
CV.24	In the depression in the centre of mentolabial groove. Above the chin.

GOVERNOR MERIDIAN

GOVERNOR MERIDIAN is an extra-ordinary meridian, controls all Yang Meridians and is on the surface of the midline and is a single meridian.

GV.1	At the tip of coccyx.
GV.2	In the hiatus of the sacrum.
GV.3	Below spinous process of the 4th lumbar vertebra.
GV.4	On the spinous process of the 2nd lumbar vertebra.
GV.6	Below the spinous process of the 12th thoracic vertebra.
GV.14	Below the spinous process of the 7th cervical vertebra (vertebra prominens).
GV.20	Centre of the head joining the apices of the two ears and sagittal suture.
GV.25	Tip of the nose.
GV.28	Philtrum — on the inner surface of the upper lip.

MERIDIANS

Fig. 55

BL.67
GB.44
SP 1
Li 1
ST 45

Nail points—foot

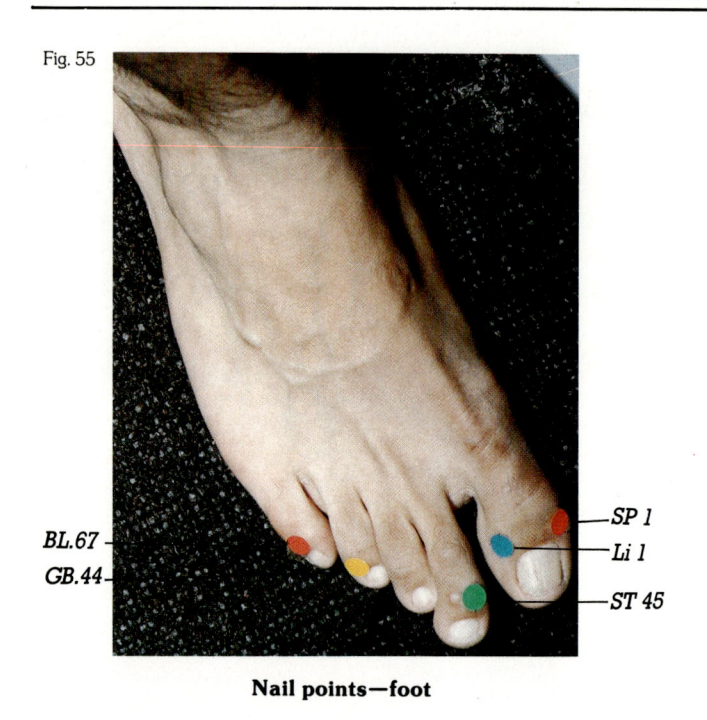

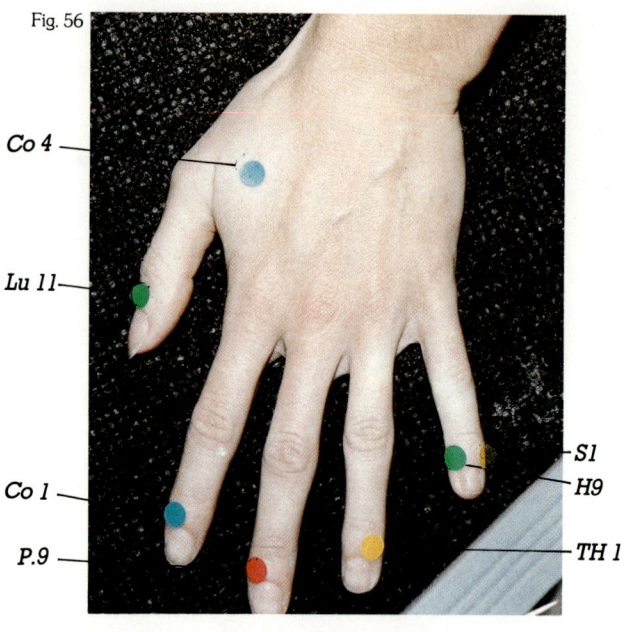

Fig. 56

Co 4
Lu 11
Co 1
P.9
S1
H9
TH 1

Nail points—hand

MEERAN'S LAWS FOR MERIDIANS

Law 1 All Meridians start or end at a Nail Point.
Law 2 In the upper limb or hand.
  (a) All Yang Meridians start at a nail point: CO.1, TH.1, S.I.1.
  (b) All Yin Meridians end at a nail point:— LU.11, P.9, H.9.
Law 3 In the lower limb or foot.
  (a) All Yang Meridians end at a nail point:— St.45, G.B.44, B.67.
  (b) All Yin Meridians start at a nail point:— Sp1, Li1, Ki1.

Two facts must be known in studying Meridians:—

1. *Cun Measurement* — is the distance between the two internal creases in the finger when the middle finger is flexed at the proximal and distal inter phalangeal joints.
2. *Nail Point* — is found by drawing a tangent to the convex border of the proximal end of the nail and joining the lateral nail fold.

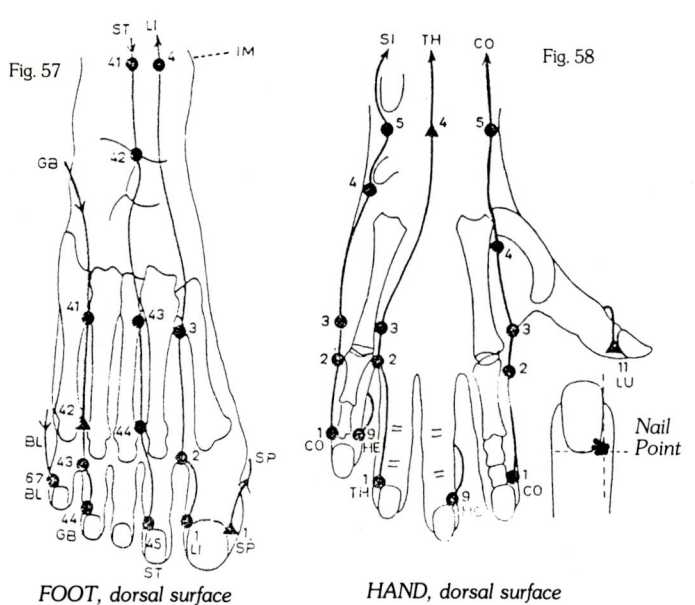

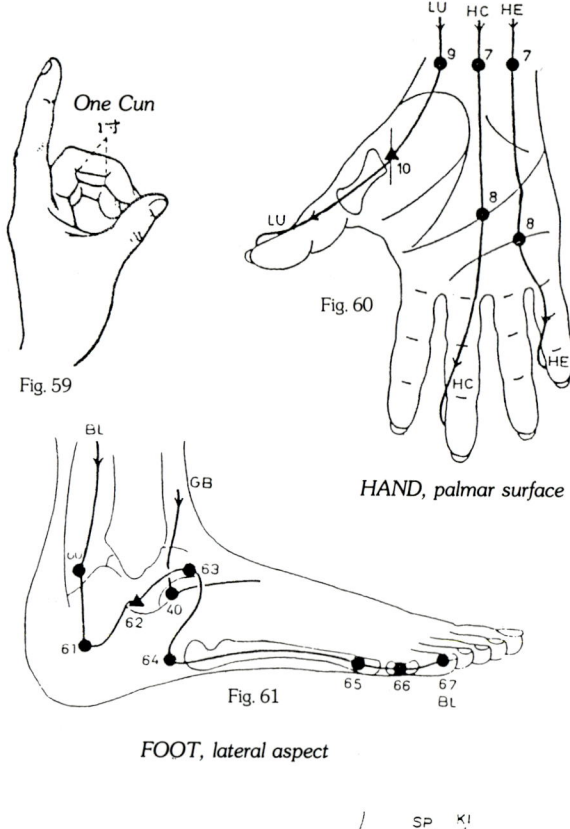

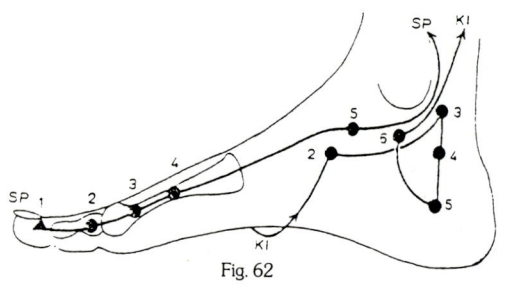

Fig. 59 — One Cun

Fig. 60

HAND, palmar surface

Fig. 57

FOOT, dorsal surface

Fig. 58

HAND, dorsal surface

Fig. 61

FOOT, lateral aspect

Fig. 62

FOOT, medial aspect

36

Pain Pathway and Gate Control Theory

1. gate Control Theory of Melzack and Wall

2. Arthritis of the Knees

3. Cervical Spondylosis

4. Lumbo-Sacral Disc Lesion

PAIN PATHWAY AND GATE CONTROL THEORY

When pain is perceived many complex mechanisms and pathways come into play. Nerve fibres at the pain source, ex. lower abdomen, transmit pulses of information to the brain at speeds determined by the thickness of the individual fibre. Large fibres conduct impulses at a faster rate than small fibres and the outcome of this is that the pulses of information reach the brain in a pattern of impulses that are separated both by space, amongst the different nerve fibres, and time. The brain's interpretation of these patterns depends on its assessment of their significance and where they come from.

In 1965, Melzack and Wall put forward the gate Control Theory to explain pain. They envisaged a mechanism rather like a butterfly valve (the gate) situated between the pain source and the brain which controls the flow of impulses to the brain. The gate, normally held ajar by a continuous stream of low level impulses along small fibres, can be opened wider by a rise in the number of large fibre impulses. When an unpleasant stimulus like a labour pain occurs the traffic along both types of fibre increases dramatically, but because the pulses travel faster in the large fibres, the initial effect is to close the pain gate.

The large fibres adapt to the increased traffic much quicker than the small fibres. Where the stimulation is prolonged, as in labour, the volume of large fibre traffic actually decreases, the gate opens and the small fibre traffic flows through, resulting in the perception of pain.

An overriding control on the system is imposed by large traffic which travels directly up the spinal column, triggering the gate to close. This control explains the apparent unawareness of pain commonly shown by games players during the excitement of a violent game. For the same reason electroacupuncture used during childbirth can block out pain. The electrical stimulation given to the hand and leg points in this large fibre sensory input, travels up to the brain to impose central control on pain perception. (Fig. 65 and 141)

Electroacupuncture has another important function during delivery. It inhibits the synthesis of prostaglandins, the body's natural pain enhancers, so giving an anti-pain effect. In birth without acupuncture, cells in the target area of the lower abdomen release a chemical (arachidonic acid) from special sites on their outer surfaces during the process of contraction. By the action of a special enzyme, prostaglandin synthetase, this chemical is converted to the pain-inducing prostaglandin.

There is another group of body chemicals that play a role in the pain process, but whereas prostaglandins are pain enhancers, these are natural pain killers, four to six times as strong as morphine. Though acupuncture prevents the release of the former, it encourages the release of the latter. These peptides, endorphin and encephalin, are made in particular areas of the brain, spinal column, and pituitary gland. Again the site of their action is the pain's target area, the lower abdomen, where they act on specific receptor sites (large molecules) on the surface of cells that are near connections (synapses). The more potent of the two is encephalin, which can be produced in preference to endorphin by using high frequency electroacupuncture of about 100 cycles per second, as in childbirth.

The three factors, gate control, prostaglandin inhibition and encephalin release are central to the success of acupuncture as a pain relief agent.

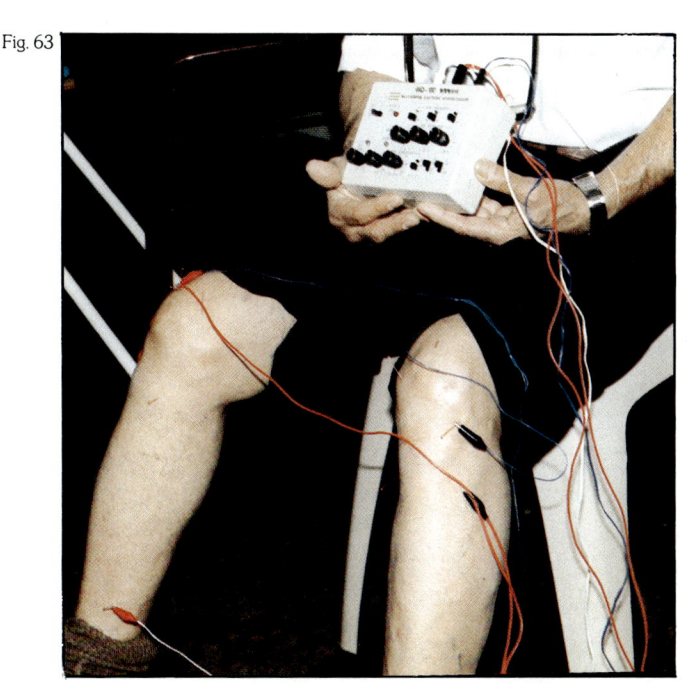

Fig. 63

Arthritis of the knees, St 36 G.B. 34. Sp6 and local tender points.

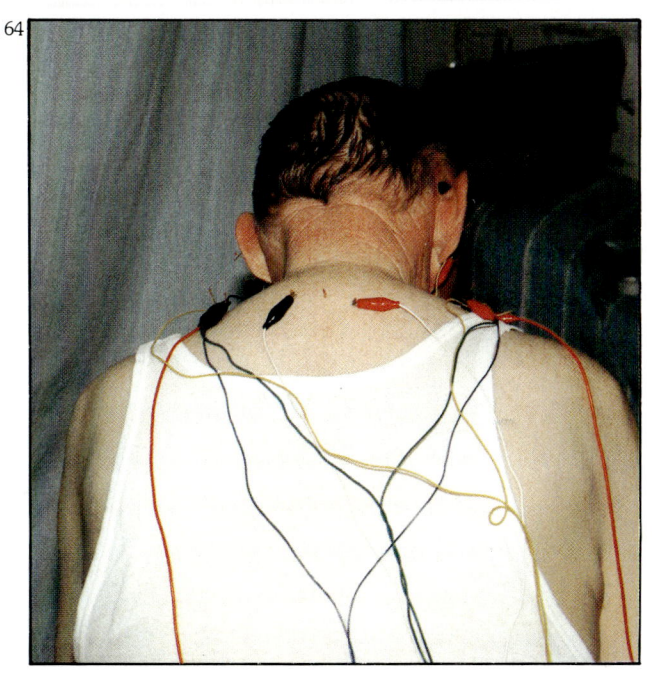

Fig. 64

Cervical-Spondylosis Bladder 11 at T1 level, Gall Bladder 21 in Supra-clavicular Fossa G.V.13 Dense Disperse Current f_1 6 f_2 20 Hertz for 40 minutes was used.

PAIN PATHWAY AND THEORY OF MELZAK AND WALL

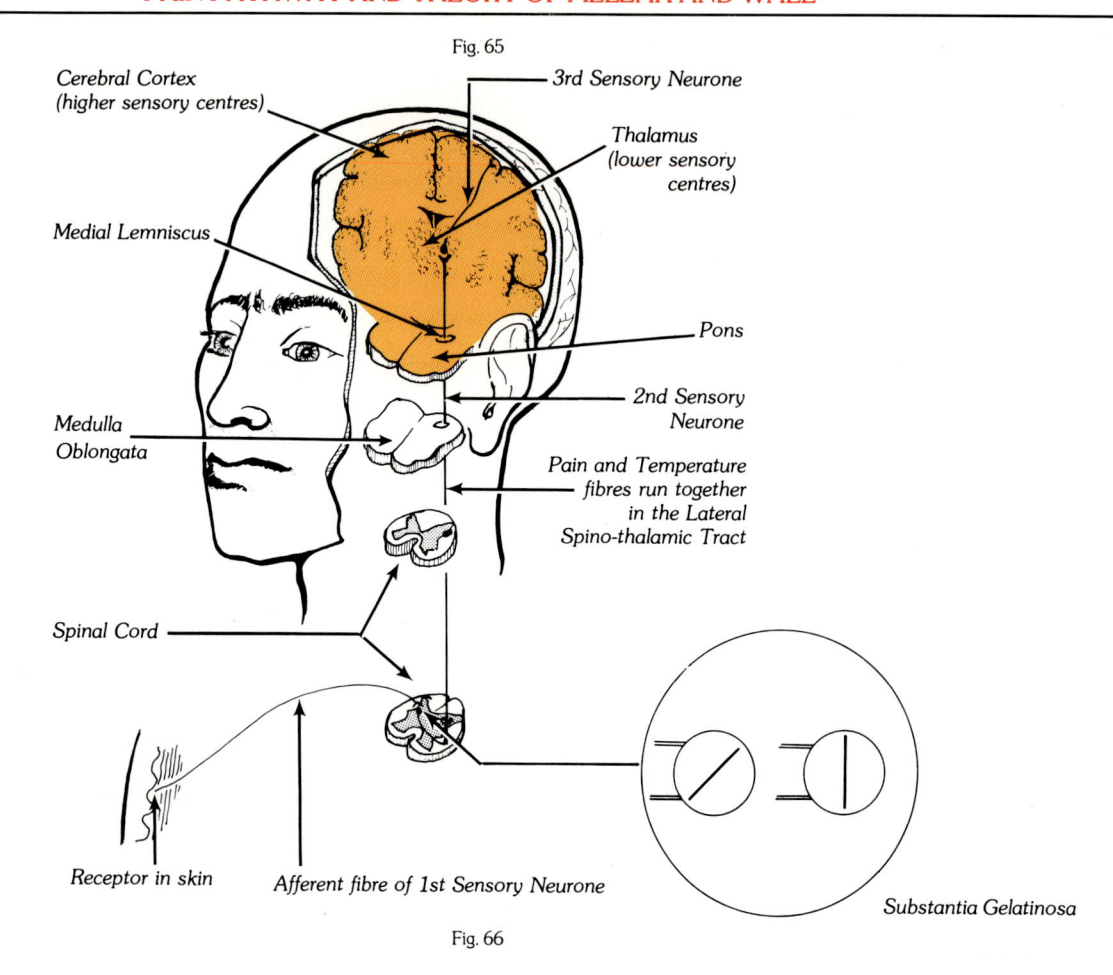

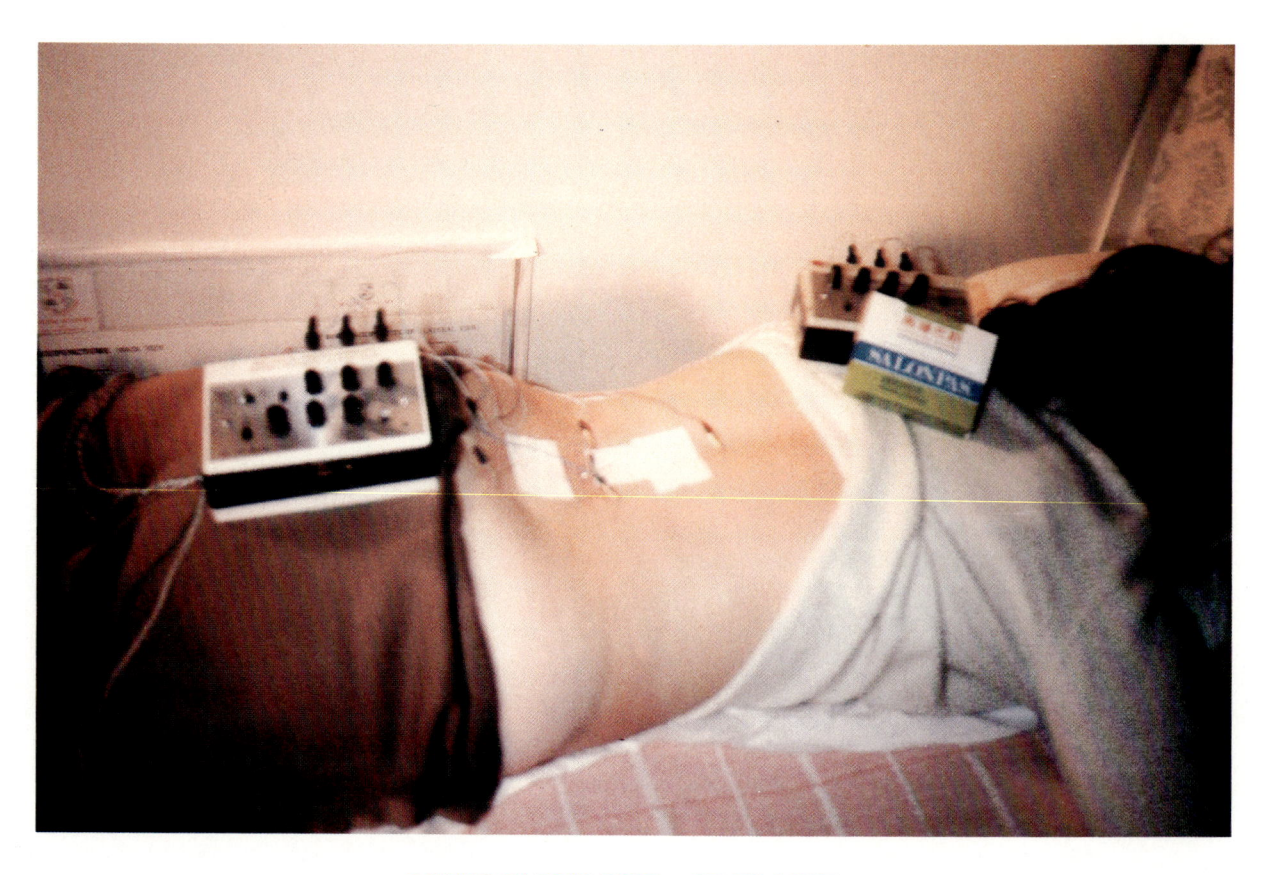

Fig. 65

- Cerebral Cortex (higher sensory centres)
- 3rd Sensory Neurone
- Thalamus (lower sensory centres)
- Medial Lemniscus
- Pons
- 2nd Sensory Neurone
- Medulla Oblongata
- Pain and Temperature fibres run together in the Lateral Spino-thalamic Tract
- Spinal Cord
- Receptor in skin
- Afferent fibre of 1st Sensory Neurone
- Substantia Gelatinosa

Fig. 66

LUMBO-SACRAL DISC — BACK-ACHE
Bladder Pts. 23, 31, 34 Bilateral B1 50 (not shown) Governor Pts. 4, & Ear Zone: Corresponding to Lumbo-Sacral spine in triangular Fossa. Electro-Acupuncture Frequency 8 and 20 Dense Disperse for 30 minutes.

Laser Therapy

1. **Principles of the Laser**

2. **Laser Machines**
    - (a) Theralaser
    - (b) Unilaser

3. **Technique of using the Laser**
    - (a) Treating Local Points
    - (b) Rectilinear Stroking
    - (c) Corona Technique

LASER THERAPY — A NEW FRONTIER

Electroacupuncture has largely superseded traditional acupuncture because it has proved to be quicker and more effective than manual manipulation. The trend towards more effective and efficient techniques has continued with the result that a new area of acupuncture has sprung up that does away with needles completely.

The new technique is laser therapy, the use of a weak laser beam to stimulate acupuncture points. It works on exactly the same principles as both traditional and electro-acupuncture, a stimulation from a source (hand/acupunctoscope/laser) is transmitted to the acupuncture point. In manual and electroacupuncture the needle is the agent of transmission; in laser therapy the beam takes the stimulation directly to the point without the need for a go-between. In this respect it may be likened to some types of moxibustion, but the similarity ends here, for the new technique is entirely painless and very quick and is simple to use.

Laser therapy means that a whole range of new patients who would not have tolerated needle insertion, can be treated safely, especially important in this category are young children. By its very nature it also ensures absolute sterility, as the skin is never broken and skin irritation is never observed at the very low strengths used. A valuable plus from the doctor's point of view is that laser therapy takes less than a third of the time needed for needling.

Let us examine the stimulation source used in laser therapy, the laser. We have probably all heard the horrific tales of blinding and scarring caused by untrained people trying to remove wrinkles and tattoos. Unfortunately these few cases have seriously blackened the laser's copy book, but the enormous potential of the correctly used laser must not go unrealised.

In order to appreciate the value of lasers in medicine we must first understand what a laser beam is and how it works. Daylight is a type of energy. It is in fact a continuous series of electromagnetic waves, with a wavelength of about a millionth of a metre, a frequency of some 500 million cycles per second and a speed of 300,000 kilometres per second. There are many other types of electromagnetic wave that are invisible to the human eye. In fact the whole spectrum stretches from long wave radio waves, through microwaves, infra red rays, visible light rays, ultra-violet rays and X-rays to very short wavelengths.

A laser beam is basically an electromagnetic wave that is loaded with far more energy than normal and it can be of many different forms, most are invisible to the human eye. The laser medium that induces this high-energy beam can be gaseous (helium/neon, argon, krypton, carbon dioxide), liquid (a dyestuff in a suitable solvent) or solid (ruby).

Two Mirror Principle of Laser Technology

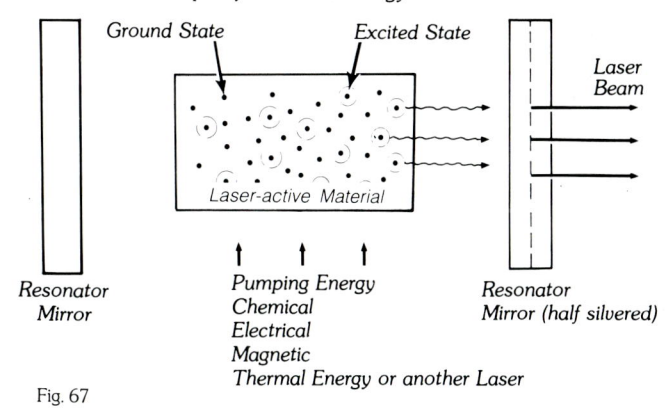

Fig. 67

All atoms and molecules (groups of atoms) give off radiation when they are excited by heat, light, electricity or some other form of energy. In a laser the molecules and atoms of the laser medium are excited in a controlled and very efficient way. Typically excited molecules release energy in very short pulses, comprising a short train of waves, and known as a wave packet or photon. In a laser all the atoms or molecules are made to produce photons of identical wavelength and the waves are all in time with each other, or in phase. Whereas in an ordinary light lamp the photons are not emitted in phase with each other and a far fewer proportion of them are excited to the highest energy status as they are in laser lamps.

Because the waves of light produced by a laser are all in phase they reinforce or amplify each other, and it is this characteristic that gave the laser its name.

Light

Amplification by

Stimulated

Emission of

Radiation

A laser produces its beam from only one end, in contrast to a normal strip light which produces light through its sides. Inside the laser photons are travelling in all directions. Apart from a small proportion of these that are lost through the side walls, most are reflected to and fro between two mirrors, one at each end of the material. One of the mirrors reflects all the photons that hit it, whereas the other has a small transparent patch through which a very fine beam of laser light can escape. The beam that comes out is a high energy parallel stream of photons of identical wavelength that can be focused accurately onto minute areas. The wavelength of the beam can be selected with great precision by adjusting the distance between the two internal mirrors.

The lasers used in acupuncture are gas-filled tubes that produce continuous rather than pulsed beams; the latter are far too strong. The helium-neon laser or theralaser (gallium diode) is a common choice. Its infra red (invisable rays) beam, emitted via a hand held pencil, has a power of two milliwatts - extremely weak when compared to the

LASER THERAPY

average 100 watt electric light bulb. The beam is just strong enough to produce thermal vibrations in human tissue and there is no need to protect the eyes.

Laser therapy involves locating the point, holding the laser pencil two to six millimetres above it and irradiating the point for 20 to 90 seconds. As well as direct irradiation of the points, the pencil can be used for stroking. This is an additional application of the laser pencil which involved specific waving and stroking movements over zones of acupuncture points.

Any condition that is suitable for electroacupuncture can also be treated by laser therapy. Complaints like trigeminal neuralgia (severe facial pain), cervical spondylosis (neck pain), backaches, migraines and nervous disorders are particularly suitable. Laser therapy is at least equal to electroacupuncture in the majority of cases. Besides this it has the added bonus of no needle insertion and therefore no pain fear, absolute sterility as the skin is never broken, the extra therapeutic potential of the stroking technique, and a reduction in treatment time of about 70 per cent.

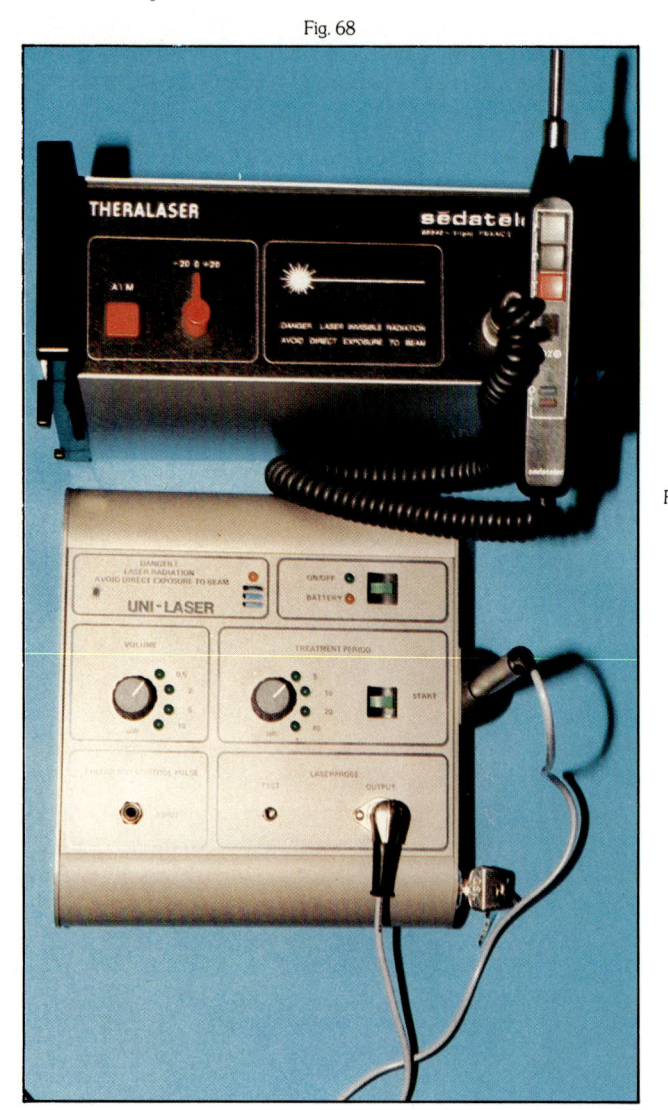

Fig. 68

Top: Theralaser   **Bottom:** Unilaser.

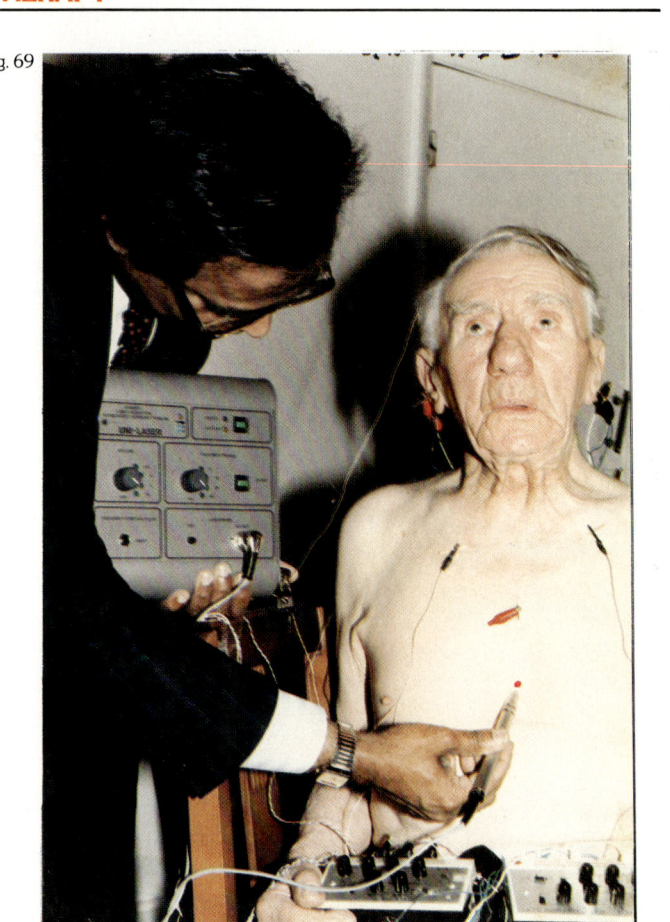

Fig. 69

Treating a patient with Unilaser and Electro-acupuncture

LASERS used in the various branches of Medicine, surgery etc. are of three types:
  Gaseous Lasers — Helium-Neon, Argon, Krypton and CO_2.
  Liquid Lasers formed mainly by dye stuffs in suitable solvent.
  Solid State Lasers — Ruby, Nd Yag laser.
  IN ACUPUNCTURE HELIUM-NEON, INFRA RED AND THERALASER ARE USED.
  The three essential physical properties of the laser are 1. Monochromaticity. 2. Coherence. 3. Maximum Parallelism.
  The laser can be used for Body Points and Ear Points.

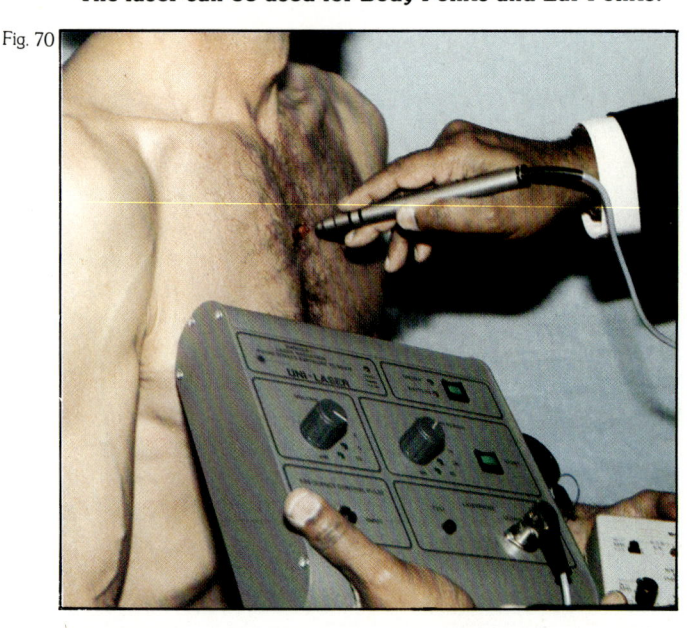

Fig. 70

1. Treating Local Points Colon 4 or Anti Aggression in Ear or CV.17. Here CV.17 is treated with the Unilaser. 10 milliwatts for 20-30 seconds per acupuncture point.

LASER THERAPY

2. Recti-linear Stroking — Cervical spine in Ear.

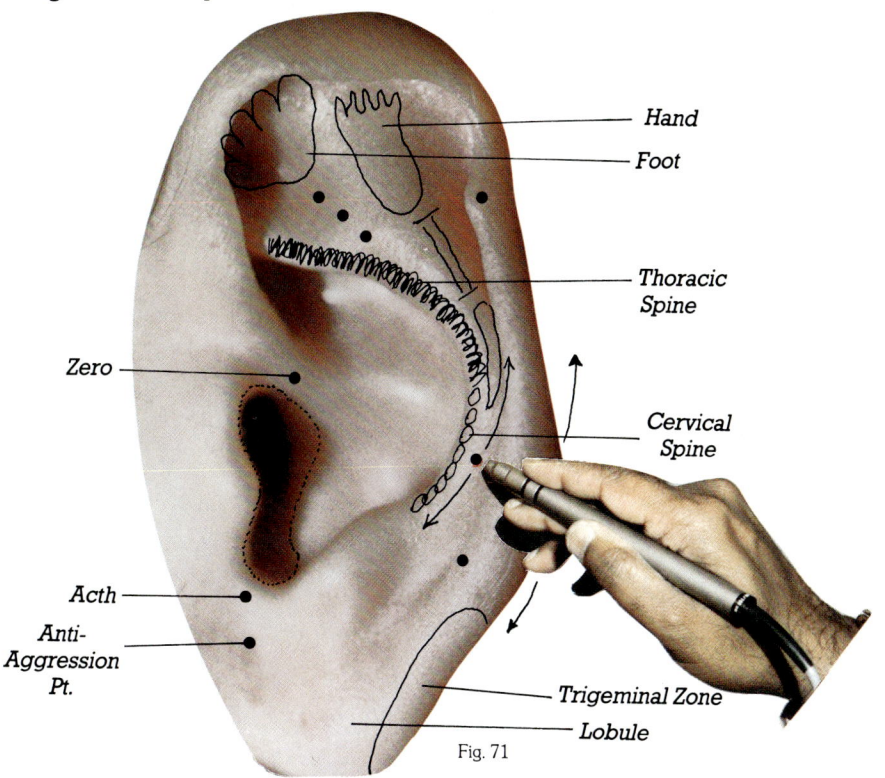

Fig. 71

In RECTI-LINEAR STROKING TECHNIQUE — Ear or Body Points can be treated. Here the cervical spine representation of the ear is being treated by stroking the area up and down as shown.

3. The CORONA-Technique.

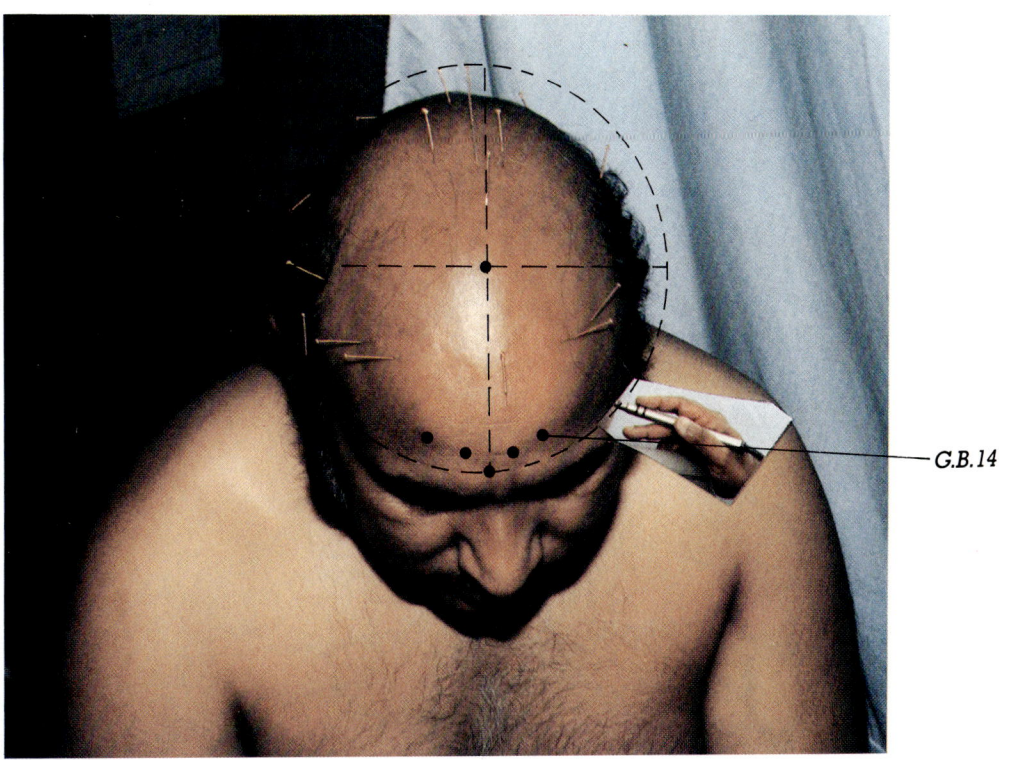

Fig. 72

In THE CORONA TECHNIQUE the pencil of the laser is taken from a point in a circular manner shown for 60-180 seconds many points belonging to different meridians can be treated in this method.
Ex. G.V. 22, G.B. 14, Bl 3, Bl 4, Bl 8, T.H. 23 etc.

Ear Acupuncture

1. Anatomy of the Ear
2. Mentally alert and special points in the ear
3. Schematic projection of Extremities, Thorax, Abdomen and points in the Lobule
4. Specific zones of the upper and lower Extremities
5. The Autonomic Nervous System
6. The projection of the Telencephalon, Motor Root of Spinal Nerves and Ear Geometry
7. Projection of the Endocrine Glands
8. Projection of the Mesencephalon and Diencephalon

EAR ACUPUNCTURE

A Chart of Auricular Acupuncture Points

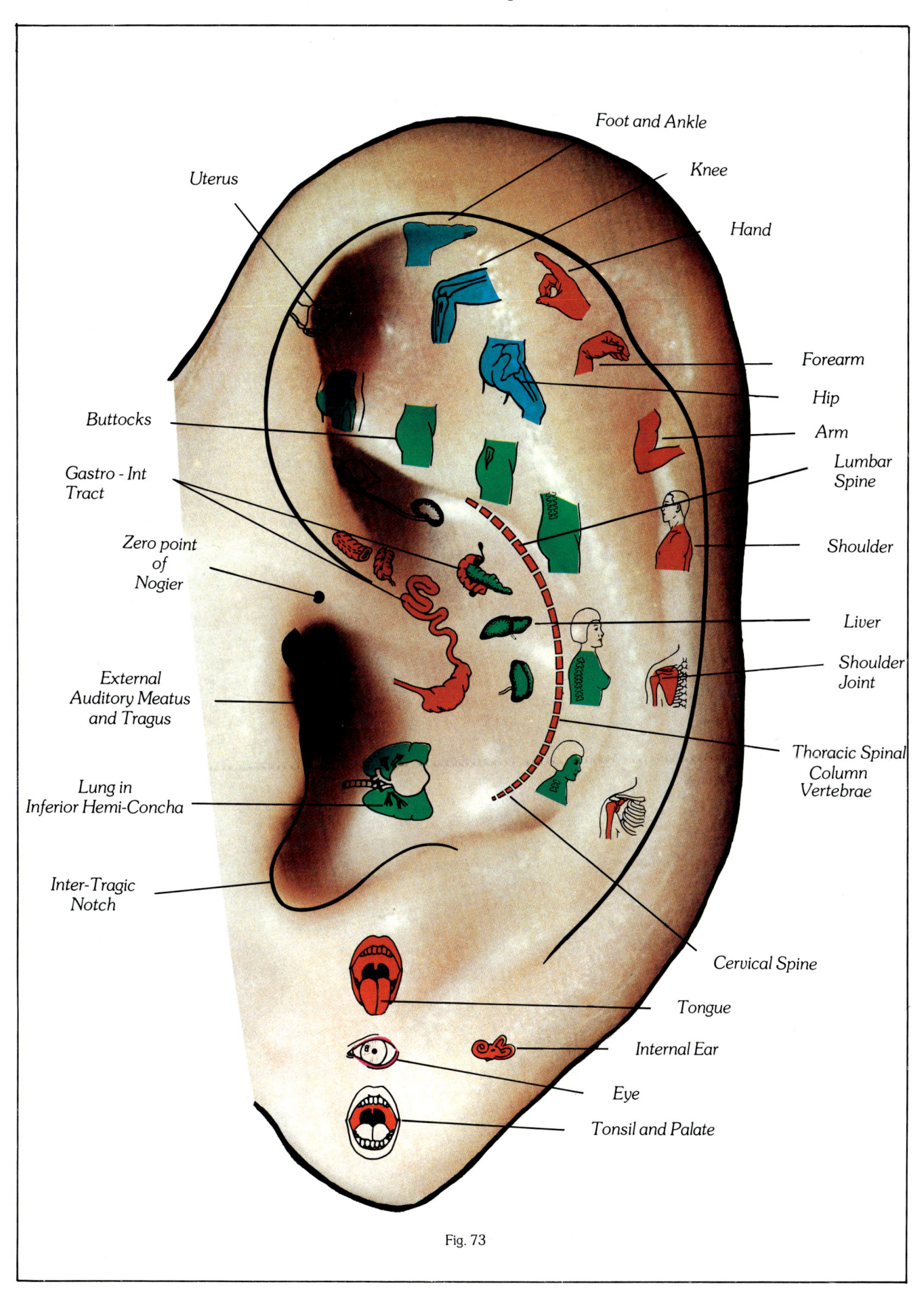

Foot and Ankle
Knee
Uterus
Hand
Forearm
Hip
Arm
Buttocks
Lumbar Spine
Gastro - Int Tract
Shoulder
Zero point of Nogier
Liver
Shoulder Joint
External Auditory Meatus and Tragus
Thoracic Spinal Column Vertebrae
Lung in Inferior Hemi-Concha
Inter-Tragic Notch
Cervical Spine
Tongue
Internal Ear
Eye
Tonsil and Palate

Fig. 73

EAR ACUPUNCTURE

Three thousand years ago the Egyptians treated backaches by touching a specific point on the ear with a red hot needle! Five minutes or so after this rather drastic treatment the offending back pains would miraculously disappear.

Such tales are the earliest record of what is today a very important and exciting area of acupuncture known as ear or auricular therapy. Totally distinct from the traditional acupuncture of the Chinese, which is based on meridians, the key to ear therapy is that there are points and zones on the ear which directly correspond to other parts of the body. Largely due to the efforts of the present day leader of ear therapy, Dr Paul Nogier of Lyon (France), the value of these points is now recognised worldwide, even by the traditional acupuncturists of China.

It is a convenient coincidence for acupuncturists that the positions of the ear's correspondence points and zones roughly conform to the position of the foetus in the womb or to an inverted man. The figure shows that points corresponding to the various parts of the face are in the fleshy lobe at the bottom of the ear whilse points corresponding to the lower limbs - (hip joint, thigh, knee joint, lower leg, ankle and foot) lie in a triangular area at the top of the ear known as the Triangular Fossa. The deep part of the centre of the ear contains points which relate to the chest and lungs in the lower portion, and to the abdominal organs like the stomach, intestine, liver, kidney and womb in the upper portion. The point for the eyes is in the centre of the lobule where many women have their ears pierced. It is a fact that fewer women than men suffer from short sight.

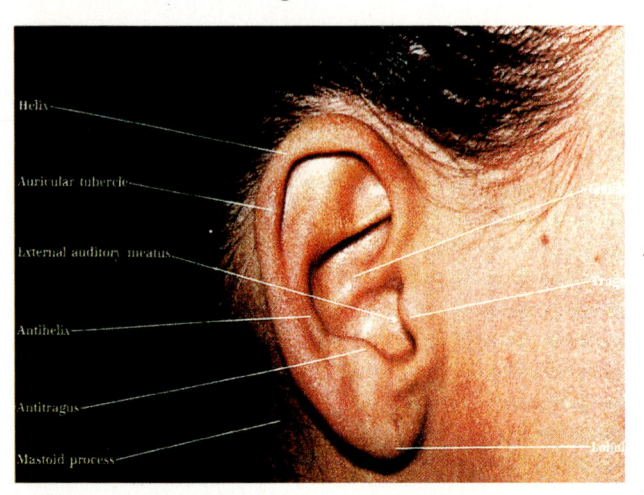

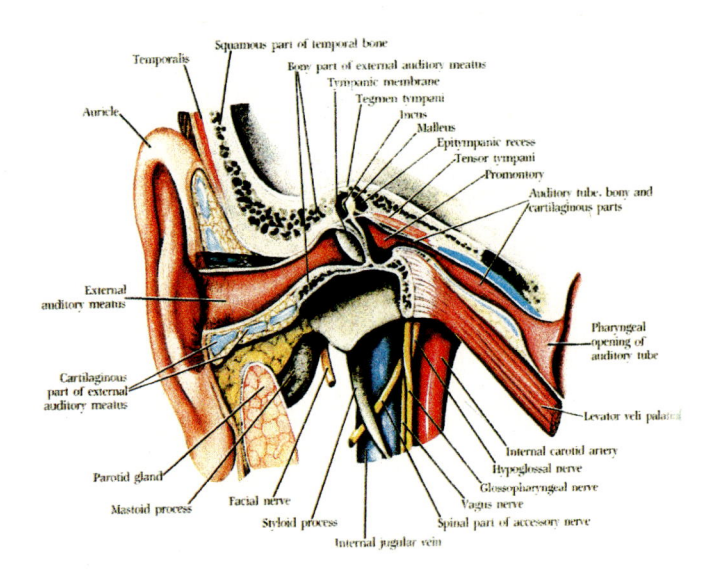

Fig. 75

The ear is made of cartilage covered with skin except at the Lobule. The cartilagious part of the ear ends at the tail of Helix (see diagram). The outer rigid parts or 'Frame' of the Pinna is formed by the Helix. This starts at the root of the Helix in the Concha (deep part of the Pinna) and proceeds upwards and then transversely. It then descends to end at the Tail of the Helix.

Below this is the Lobule — the soft part of the Pinna with no cartilage. The upper part of the pinna is divided into the superficial part which forms a triangle bounded by the Helix at the base and the inferior and superior crus of the Anthelix. The Apex of this triangle is at the level of the

Fig. 74

There are 292 known ear points and many of these have been discovered by Dr Nogier. Examples of the numerous conditions that can be treated by needling ear points or a combination of ear and body points are as follows:—

Nervous Tension, Obesity, Smoking, Phobias, Insomnia, Migraine, Headaches, Impotence and Frigidity, Psychosexual Disorders, Arthritis (spine, hip, knee, shoulder), Trigeminal Neuralgia, Skin and Allergic Disorders.

It is important that before Auricular Therapy is studied, the student should know the structure of the Auricle (Pinna) thoroughly.

Fig. 76

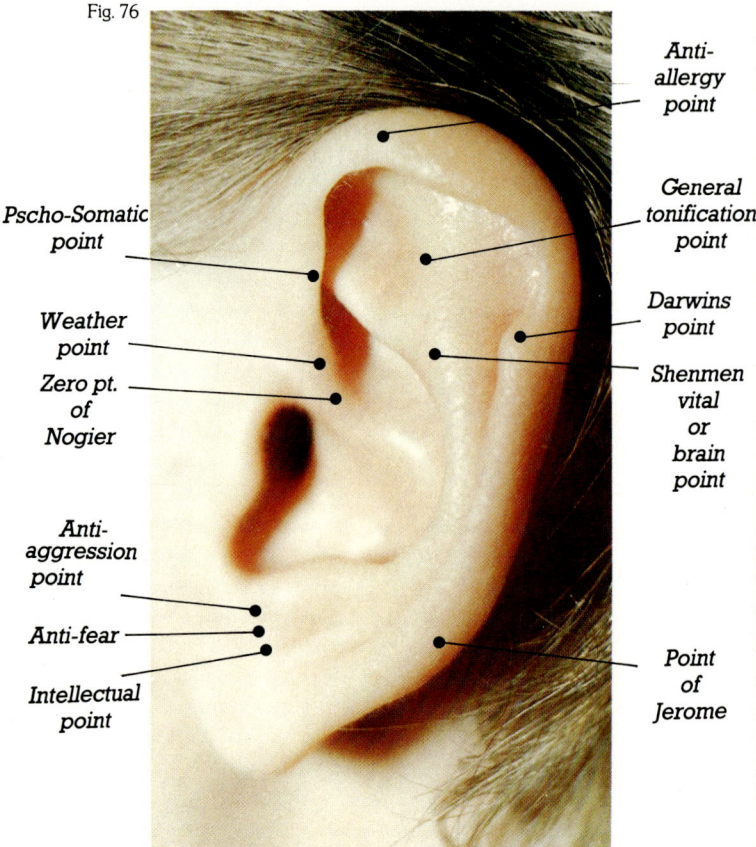

Mentally alert and special points of the ear.

EAR ACUPUNCTURE

body of the Anthelix and the hip joint is situated at the apex. This triangular area, which is anterior to the upper crus, is a depression and is referred to as the Triangular Fossa.

Posterior to the Triangular Fossa is the Scaphoid Fossa, which is formed by the upper crus of Anthelix, the posterior border of the body of the Helix and a line drawn obliquely from the anterior crus of the Anthelix, situated in this fossa is the correspondence point of the hand. Also, projecting into this fossa is the tubercle of the Helix. The correspondence points for the vertebral column are situated in the posterior border of the body of the Anthelix.

The Concha is the deep part of the Pinna. Anteriorly, it is formed by Tragus; just posterior is the External Auditory Meatus. There are many imporatant corresponding points in the Concha. If the root of the Helix is extended posteriorly, it divides the Concha into Superior Hemi-Concha and the Inferior Hemi Concha. The points for respiratory systems are in Inferior Hemi Concha, and the Gastro-Intestinal System is in the Superior Hemiconcha.

SCHEMATIC PROJECTION OF THE EXTREMITIES AND THE SPINE

In the triangular fossa is represented the lower extremities namely the foot, ankle, leg (tibia, fibula), knee joint, thigh (femur) and hip joint. At the apex of the triangular fossa is the point which is referred to as Shenmen which is also called the brain or vital point and has a relaxing effect on the body.

In the scaphoid fossa is represented the upper limb namely hand, forearm with radius and ulna, the arm with humerus clavicle and scapula.

Also represented in this diagram is the spine which is divided into 7 cervical, 12 thoracic, 5 lumbar, sacrum and coccyx. The root of the helix when prolonged backwards cuts the 3rd cervical vertebra in the anti-helix. The 12 ribs are also shown with the heart situated in the 4th and 5th thoracic vertebrae.

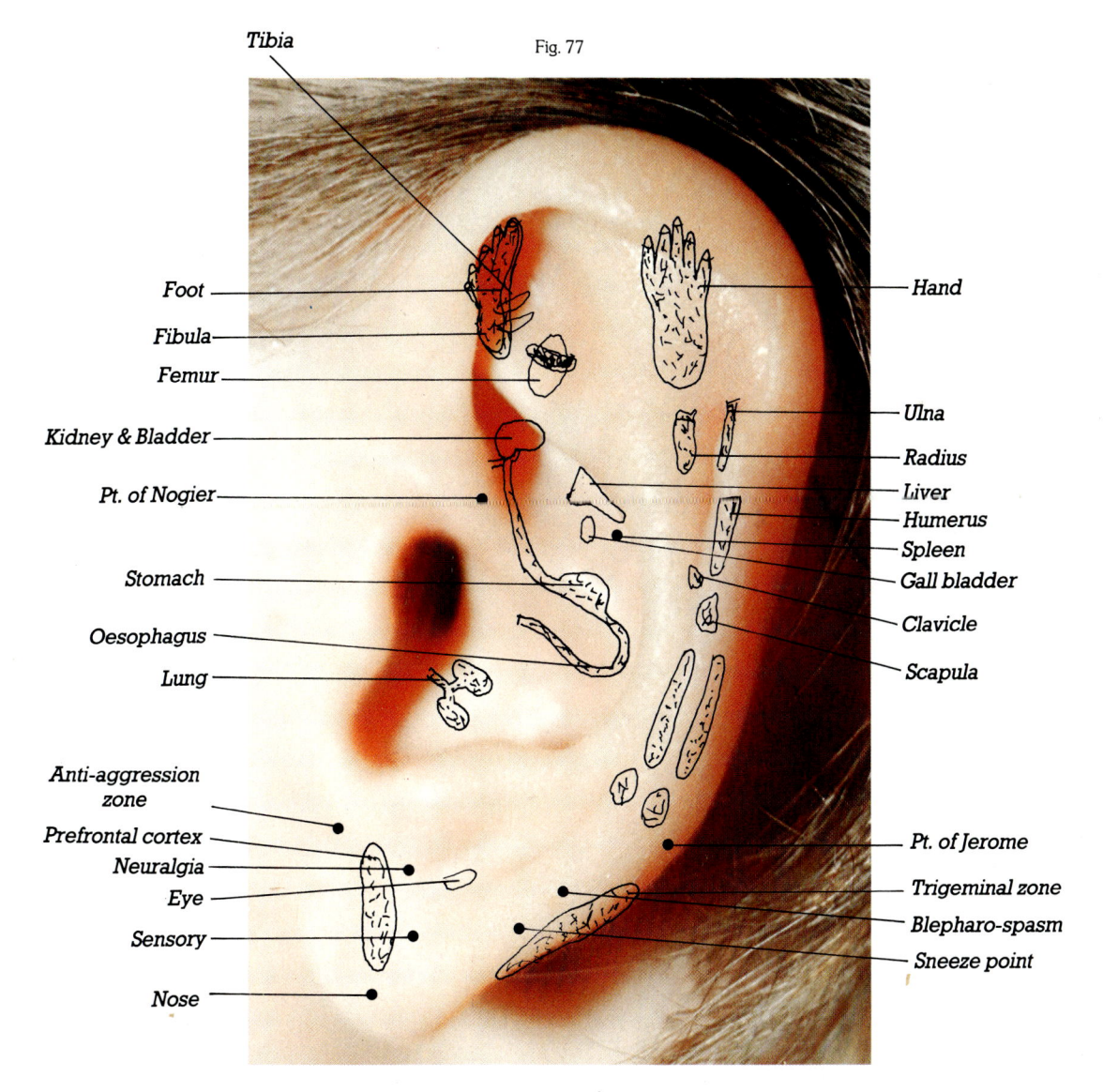

Fig. 77

Schematic projection of extremities, thorax, abdomen and points in the lobule.

EAR ACUPUNCTURE

SPECIFIC ZONE OF THE UPPER AND LOWER EXTREMITIES

This picture shows the upper and lower extremities with gluteal muscles, sciatic nerve. The sciatic nerve was the point used by the early Egyptians by cauterising this point to relieve backache and pain in the lower limbs.

Fig. 78

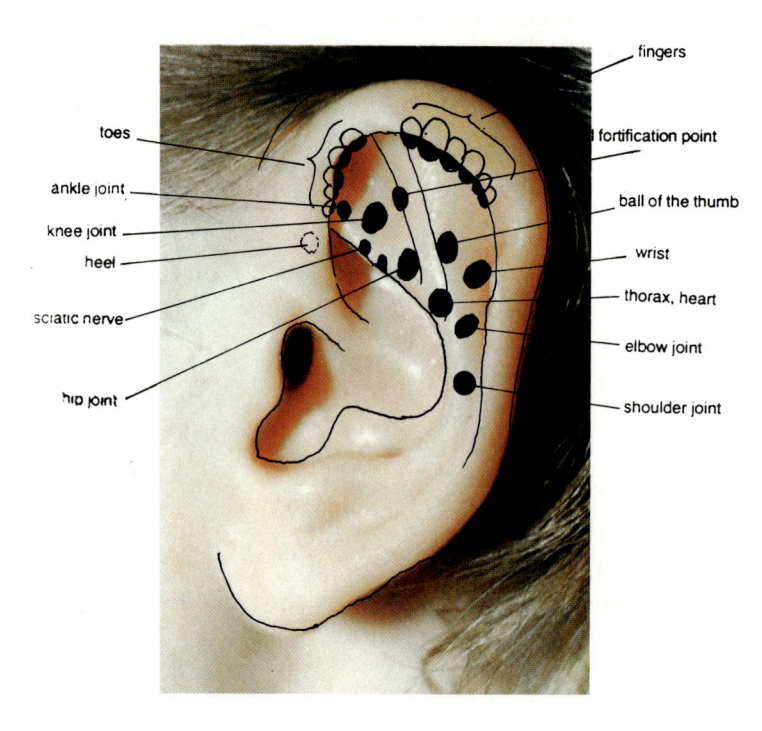

Specific zones of the upper and lower extremities

Fig. 79

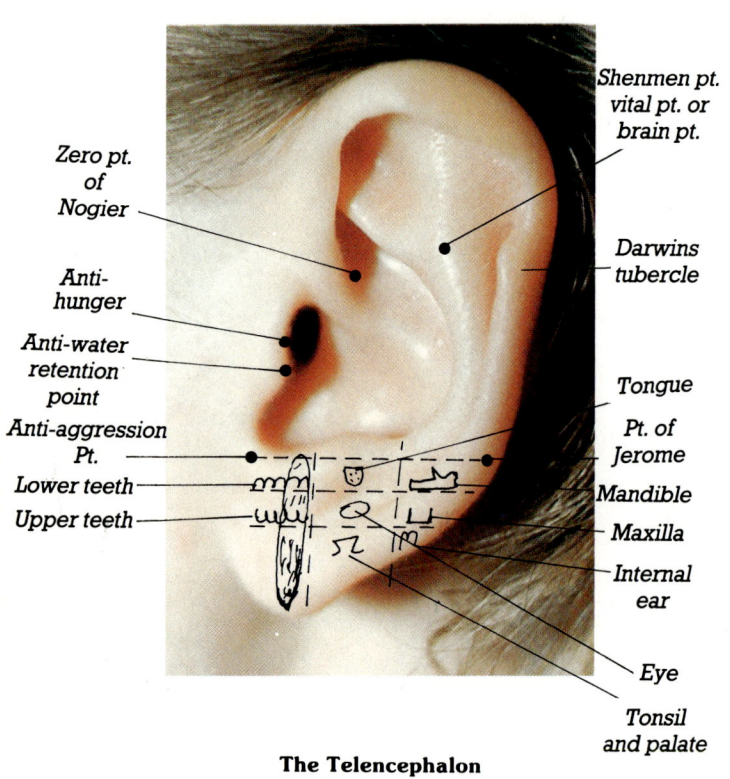

The Telencephalon

ZONES OF THE CRANIAL BONES, SINUSES, MAXILLA, MANDIBLE AND MUSCLES OF THE NECK

The Telencephalon is represented in the antitragus with the frontal lobe and bone behind which is the temperoparietal lobe and bone and occipital lobe and bone. At the foot of the Anti-tragus when the anterior

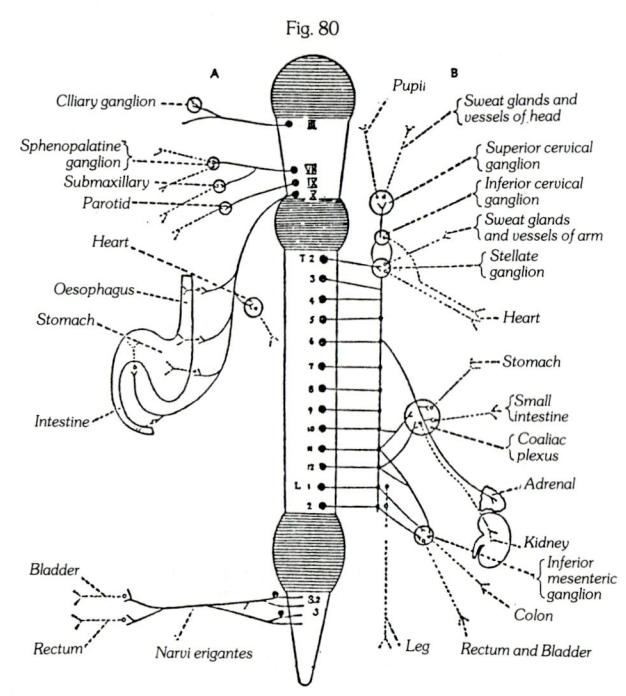

Fig. 80

Plan of autonomic nervous system. The thoracolumbar outflow is separated from the bulbosacral outflow by the cervical and lumbar limb enlargements of the cord. Preganglionic fibres are shown as uninterrupted lines, post-ganglionic fibres as broken lines. A, Parasympathetic; B, Sympathetic. (Re-drawn from 'The Sympathetic Nervous System in Desease', by W. Langdon Brown).

Fig. 81

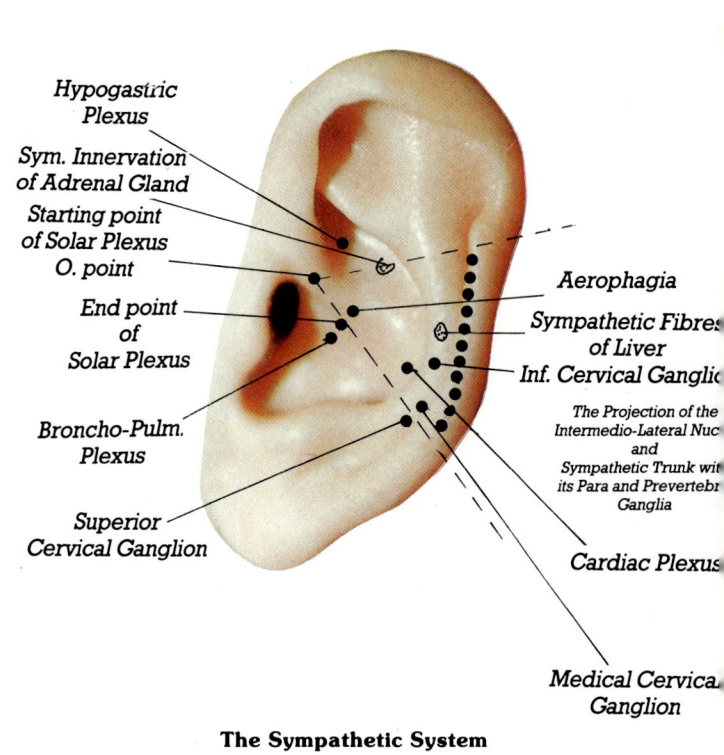

The Sympathetic System

EAR ACUPUNCTURE

THE PROJECTION OF THE TELENCEPHALON

The various projections of the telencephalon as shown in the figure are self-explanatory. Emphasis must be made to the trigeminal zone and the prefrontal cortex as the former is used in Trigeminal Neuralgia and the latter in emotional disturbances. The other part that must be emphasised is the sensory zone namely, the auditory zone, rectangular area below the antitragus which is used in tinnitus and menieres syndrome.

with courtesy - Helmut Kropej M.D.

Fig. 82

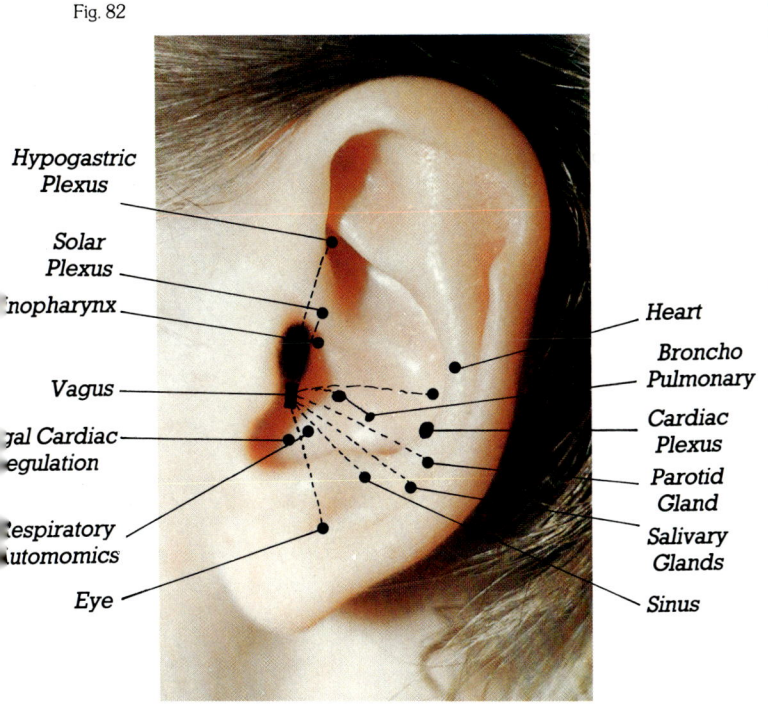

Parasympathetic System

1. The Projection of the Telencephalon
2. Motor Root of Spinal Nerves
3. Ear Geometry

Fig. 83

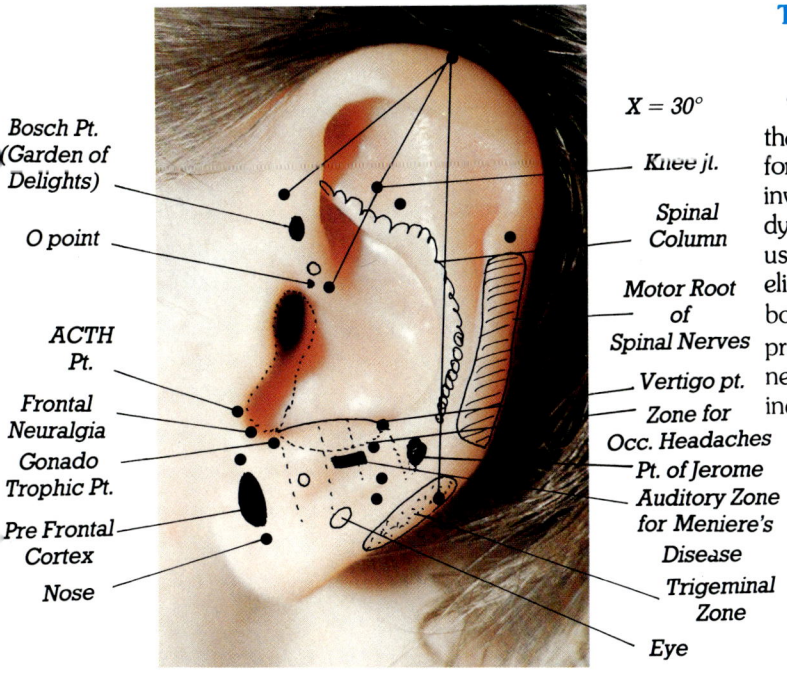

OAB is the marginal line

Fig. 84

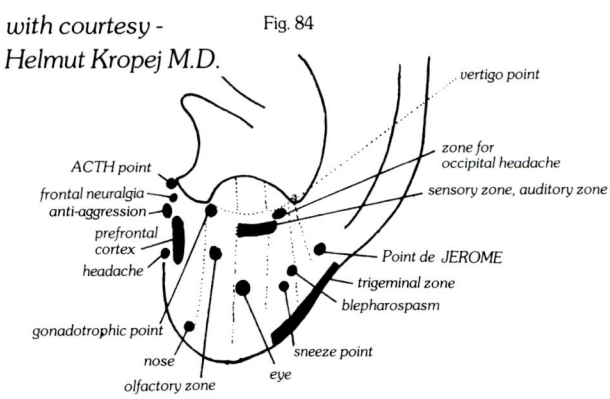

The Projection of the Telencephalon

Overall view of the projection of the diencephalon and mesencephalon in the region of the horizontal plane of the inferior hemiconcha (foot of the concha). (The tragus bent forwards, the antitragus bent downwards

SPECIAL ZONES IN THE PROJECTION OF THE DI AND MESENCEPHALON (TRAGUS BENT FORWARDS, ANTITRAGUS OUTWARDS

There is a zone under the external auditory meatus for the mesencaphalon which is for controlling muscle tone for the treatment of Parkinson's disease, Chorea and any involuntary movements. Below that is a region for dyspareunia. Also there is the thalamus point which is used for the treatment of tics and also to alleviate or eliminate all unilateral, usually homolateral pain in the body. By needling the thalamus point systolic blood pressure can be regulated. To lower blood pressure gold needle must be used. The thalamus point is contraindicated in pregnancy.

Fig. 85

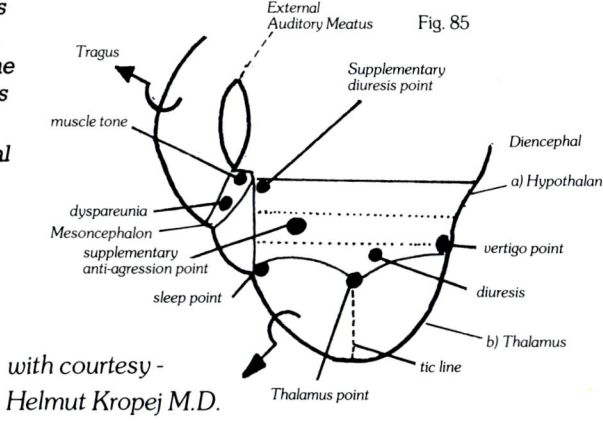

with courtesy - Helmut Kropej M.D.

Special zones in the projection of the diencephalon and mesencephalon (tragus bent forwards, antitragus downwards)

and posterior projections are joined by a line there is the frontal sinus in front, the ethmoidal sinus in the middle and the sphenoidal sinus posteriorly. Posterior to the anti-helix in the lower part are the paravertebral and ventral muscles of the neck. Below this is the maxilla and mandible, and between the two is the temporomandibular joint.

EAR ACUPUNCTURE

Projection of the Endocrine Glands Endocrine Acupuncture Points.

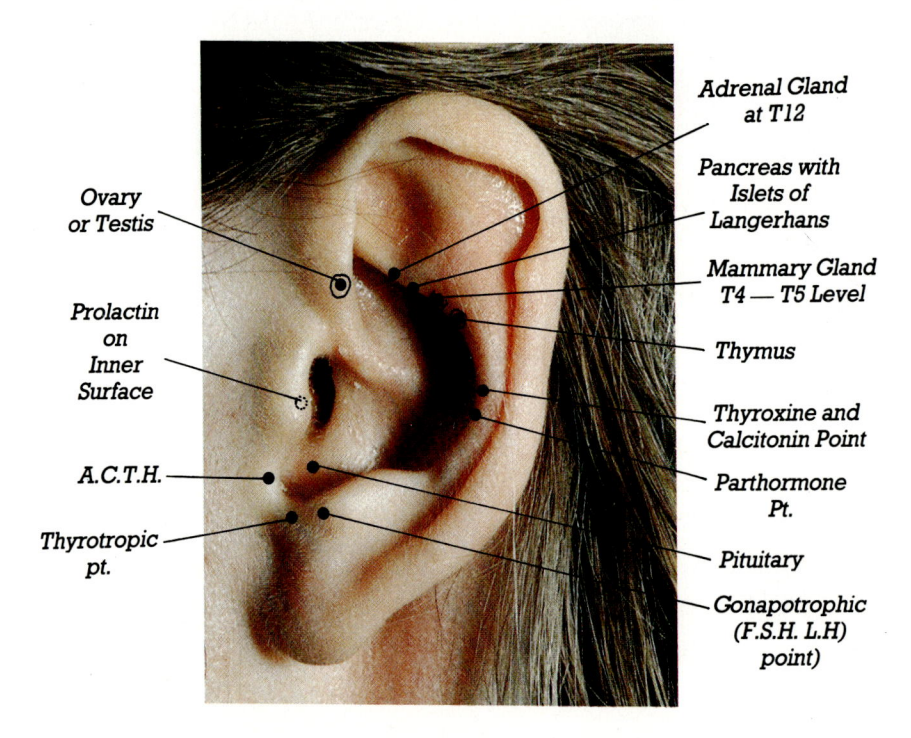

Labels on ear diagram:
- Ovary or Testis
- Prolactin on Inner Surface
- A.C.T.H.
- Thyrotropic pt.
- Adrenal Gland at T12
- Pancreas with Islets of Langerhans
- Mammary Gland T4 — T5 Level
- Thymus
- Thyroxine and Calcitonin Point
- Parthormone Pt.
- Pituitary
- Gonapotrophic (F.S.H. L.H) point)

Fig. 86

THE ENDOCRINE GLANDS

These are the ductless glands which produces the hormones of the body.

The pituitary gland which consists of the anterior and posterior lobes. The anterior lobe is developed from Rathkes Pouch — which is of ectodermal cells and it has three types of cells:— The Acidophil Cell which produces growth hormone and prolactin. The Basophil Cell produces:— 1. The Gonado-Trophic hormones (F.S.H. and L.H.) 2. The Thyrotrophic Hormone which acts on the thyroid gland to produce Thyroxine (T4) and adreno-corticotrophic hormone which acts on the adrenal cortex to produce hydrcortisone. The chromophobe cell produces the melonocyte stimulating hormone and possibly A.C.T.H. The posterior lobe of the pituitary gland produces oxytocin, and anti-diuretic hormone which acts on the distal tubules of the kidney. The other endocrine glands are shown in the diagram.

THE ENDOCRINE POINTS

The prolactin point is situated on the medial surface of the tragus. The ACTH point is situated in the anterior part just above the anti-aggression point. In the intertragic notch is the thyrotrophic point. In the gonadotrophic point which is used in sub-fertility is in the posterior part of the anti-tragus (Figs. 84, 86, 95). At the apex of the triangle in the inner surface is the adrenal gland at the level of the 12th thoracic vertebra. The mammary gland or breast is at the level of the 5th thoracic vertebra. The thyroid gland is at the level of the 6th and 7th cervical vertebrae. On the ascending branch of the helix is the ovary. Just below the external auditory meatus is the pituitary gland which in the past Landgon Brown called it the 'Leader of the Endocrine Orchestra' but in the present day it is the hypothalamus that should be considered the 'Leader of the Endocrine Orchestra' because it controls hormones through the pituitary gland by the releasing hormones produced by the Hypothalamus. (Fig. 151 Page 72)

The releasing hormones are produced by the hypothalamus which act on the pituitary gland which produces the respective hormones.

Diagrams to show the position of the chief endocrine organs in the body.

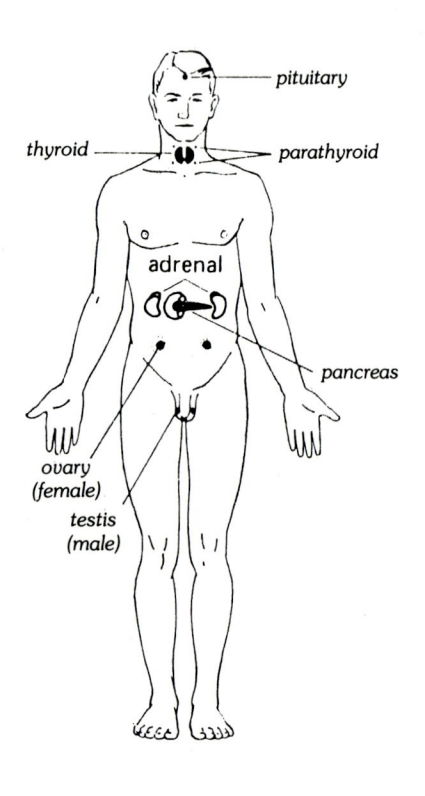

Labels on body diagram:
- pituitary
- thyroid
- parathyroid
- adrenal
- pancreas
- ovary (female)
- testis (male)

Fig. 87

Assesment and Management of Patients for Acupuncture Therapy

Guidelines

1. History

2. Examination

3. Investigations

4. Diagnosis

5. Working out Formula or Prescription

6. Positions used for Patients having Acupuncture Treatment

ASSESSMENT AND MANAGEMENT OF PATIENTS FOR ACUPUNCTURE THERAPY

GUIDELINES FOR THERAPY

In dealing with patient with whatever condition that has to be treated, PROVIDED the patient is suited to be treated with Body Acupuncture, Ear Acupuncture, Moxibustion or Laser Acupuncture it is extremely important that the following steps be adopted.

MEDICAL HISTORY

The patient's history must be taken very accurately. This should include the present complaint in detail, any past history of any illness or admission to hospital, whether any operations have been performed etc. ALL DETAILS MUST BE OBTAINED. A GOOD CLINICIAN WILL ARRIVE AT SOME FORM OF DIAGNOSIS AND WILL GET SOME IDEA OF MANAGEMENT ON A GOOD HISTORY ALONG. The next step is a thorough PHYSICAL EXAMINATION.

PHYSICAL EXAMINATION

It is essential that not only the part or system involved be examined but ALL SYSTEMS SHOULD BE EXAMINED.

INVESTIGATIONS

1. BLOOD TESTS — Haemoglobin, E.S.R., Blood Count, Serum Electrolytes, Blood Sugar, Lipid Profile including Serum Cholesterol, Serum Uric Acid.
2. LIVER FUNCTION TESTS, KIDNEY FUNCTION TESTS and other relevant ENDOCRINE FUNCTION TESTS if indicated should be performed.

RADIOLOGY

1. PLAIN X-RAYS — Chest, Abdomen, Skull, Sinuses, Bones and Joints to exclude any Pathology.
2. SPECIAL X-RAYS — Intra-venous — Urogram, Cholecystogram, etc., depending on the condition of the patient and to which system the clinician must concentrate his attention.
3. BARIUM MEAL, BARIUM ENEMA — In respect of the Gastro-Intestinal tract.
4. ULTRASOUND EXAMINATION.

Positions used for patients having Acupuncture therapy

5. ENDOSCOPY - Bronchoscopy, Oesophagoscopy, Gastroscopy, Sigmoidoscopy, Colonoscopy, Arthroscopy, Cystoscopy.
6. LUNG FUNCTION TESTS, E.C.G. and ANGIOGRAPHY, ECHO CARDIOGRAM.
7. PANCREATIC FUNCTION TESTS and E.R.C.P.
8. SKELETAL SURVEY if indicated.
9. ANY OTHER TESTS that may be required depending on the patient.
10. COMPUTERISED AXIAL TOMOGRAPHY (C.A.T. SCANS).

IT IS IMPORTANT TO EMPHASISE THAT IN A PARTICULAR PATIENT ALL THE ABOVE INVESTIGATIONS MAY NOT BE NECESSARY BUT THE CLINICIAN MUST DECIDE WHAT INVESTIGATION IS NECESSARY FOR THAT PARTICULAR PATIENT AS MANY ARE INVASIVE AND WILL BE UNNECESSARY FOR A PARTICULAR PATIENT.

THE MOST IMPORTANT FACTOR IS TO SELECT THE RIGHT PATIENT FOR THIS FORM OF THERAPY — IN OTHER WORDS, THE DIAGNOSIS OF THE CONDITION MUST BE ACCURATE.

TO SUMMARISE:—

1. HISTORY
2. EXAMINATION
3. INVESTIGATIONS
4. DIAGNOSIS
5. WORK OUT FORMULA OR PRESCRIPTION
6. TREATMENT (A) BODY POINTS
   (B) EAR POINTS
   (C) EXTRA POINTS
7. ELECTRO-ACUPUNCTURE, LASER THERAPY, MOXA IS USED ACCORDINGLY.

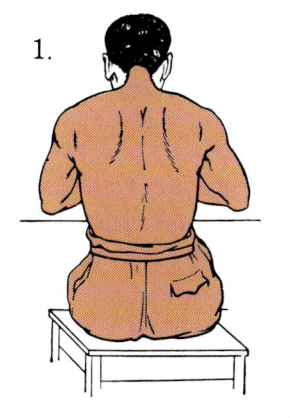

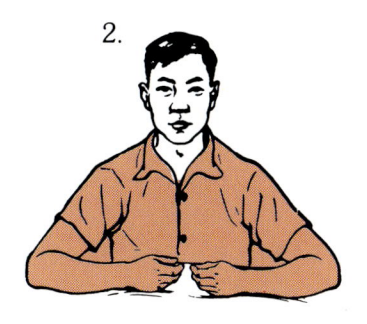

1.

2.

Fig. 88

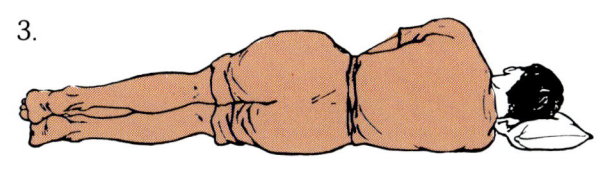

3.

Fig. 89

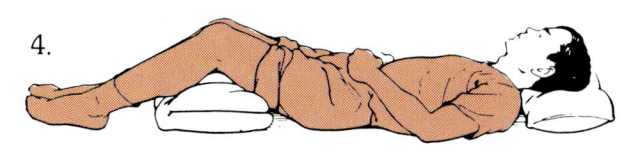

4.

Fig. 90

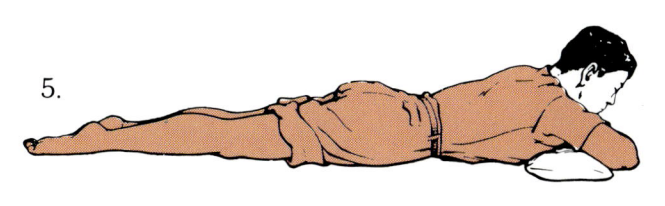

5.

Fig. 91

Treatment of Pain and Disease

1. Migraine

2. Acupuncture points for pain in face - using body points and ear points.

3. Acupuncture points for pain in lower limb and foot.

TREATMENT OF PAIN AND DISEASE

In theory any disease or pain can be treated with acupuncture, but in practice some must be dealt with by surgery. Determining the suitability of the condition for acupuncture therapy is crucial, this is why the initial diagnosis of the patient is so important.

Some common complaints that respond well include breathing problems like bronchitis and asthma; digestive tract troubles like ulcers, diarrhoea and constipation; reproductive conditions like impotence, premature ejaculation and abnormal bleeding of the womb; and nervous system complaints such as vertigo, neuralgia, sciatica and neuritis. It is also effective for hypertension, headaches, migraines, obesity and arthritis.

If, after careful diagnosis, the doctor finds the patient suitable for acupuncture, he selects the points to be needled according to the Five Element System and Ko Cycle, so deriving a specific formula for treatment (a prescription).

Pain, depending on the type, severity and location, is treated by needling points on the legs and feet. For migraine, trigeminal neuralgia or sinusitis, it is necessary to use points on the face, foot, ear and arm. Therapy for conditions like backache, arthritis, rheumatoid, osteo-arthritis involves points at the base of the spine, points on the inside and back of the legs and a single point on the ear.

There are several ways of applying these formulae. The doctor can use traditional therapy, by twirling or tapping gold or silver needles at the relevant points, or he can use electroacupuncture, the latter is preferable and gives excellent results.

If the specific formula is not suited to needling, as in some conditions of hypofunction (excess Yin), the acupuncturist can use thermal therapy (moxibustion). An example is asthma, here the overactive respiratory system is treated either by dispersing energy in the Lung meridian or alternatively stimulating the corresponding Colon meridian. A new alternative to both electroacupuncture and moxibustion is laser therapy.

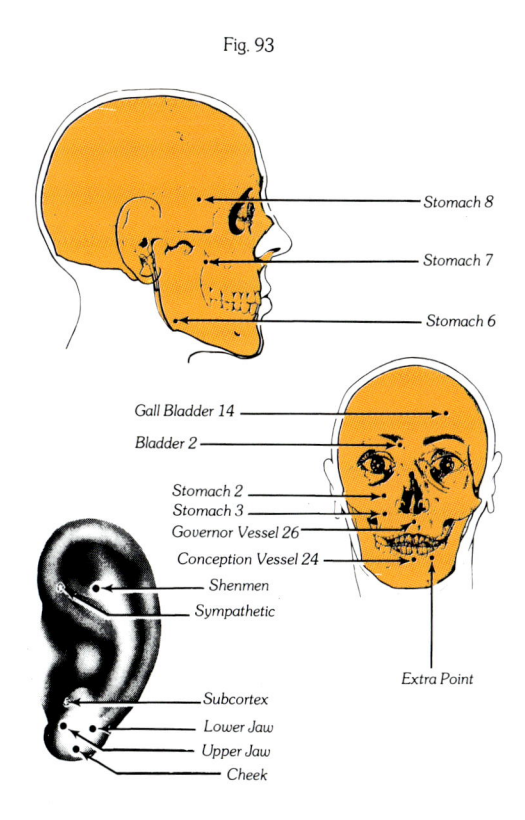

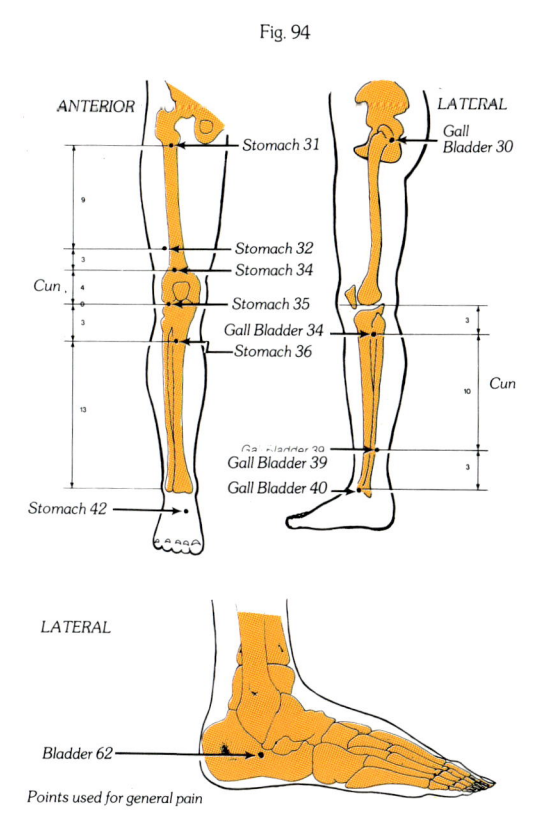

Fig. 93

Fig. 92

MIGRAINE: Body Points BL_2 St_2 GB_1 TH_{23} Bilateral CO_4

Ear Points: Anti Aggression
Trigeminal Zone } Both
Shenmen } Ears

Electroacupuncture is used 6-8 Hertz
Treatment Time 20-30 minutes
Sessions one or more weekly depending on progress.

Fig. 94

Points used for general pain

61

Orthopaedics and Rheumatology

1. Causes of Cervical and Lumbo-Sacral Pain and Sciatica
2. Cervical Spondylosis
3. Lumbo-Sacral Disc Lesion
4. Neck pain and Inter-Scapular pain
5. Burning pain, 5th Lumbar Vertebra and Sacrum
6. Rheumatoid Arthritis
8. Arthritis of the Shoulder
9. Arthritis of the Wrist
10. Carpal Tunnel Syndrome

Cervical Spine and Thoracic Inlet
Causes of Cervical Pain

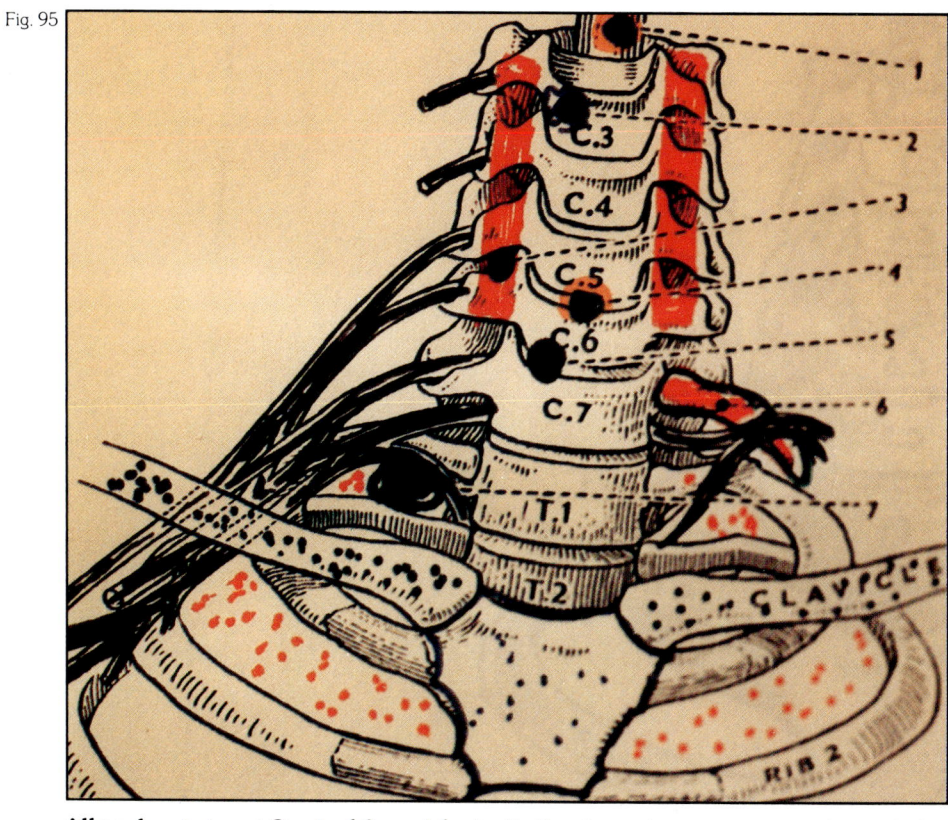

Fig. 95

1. Tumour of Spinal Cord
2. Tumour of Spinal Column
3. Tumour of Nerve Root
4. Disc Lesion (Cervical Spondylosis)
5. Osteoartrosis
6. Cervical Rib
7. Tumour of Thoracic Outlet

DIAGNOSIS
1. History. 2. Examination
3. Investigations relevant to condition see p. regarding assessment of patients

All neck pain is not Cervical Spondylosis. 8 other important causes must be excluded.

1. Tumour of Spinal Cord 2. Tumour of Spinal Column 3. Tumour of Nerve Root 4. Disc Lesion (Cervical Spondylosis)
5. Osteoarthrosis 6. Cervical Rib 7. Tumour of Thoracic Outlet.

DIAGNOSIS:
1. History 2. Examination 3. Investigations relevant to conditions - see guidelines regarding assessment of Patients. P.57

Lumbo-Sacral Spine and Pelvis   Causes of Lower Back Pain

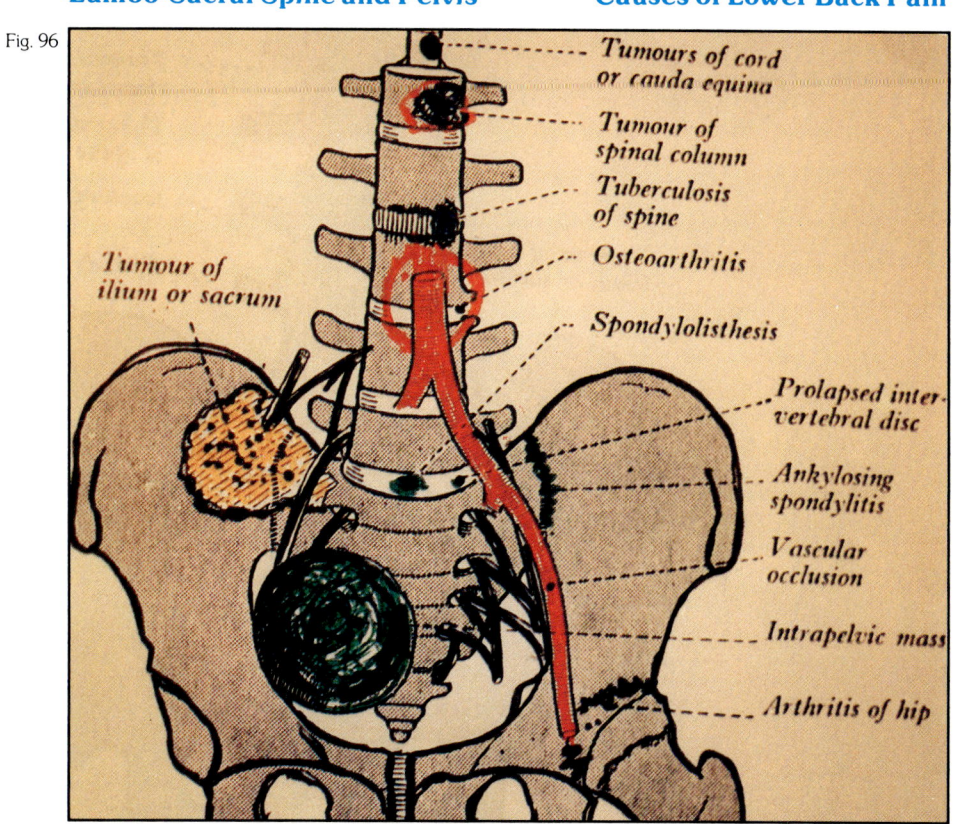

Fig. 96

- Tumours of cord or cauda equina
- Tumour of spinal column
- Tuberculosis of spine
- Osteoarthritis
- Spondylolisthesis
- Prolapsed intervertebral disc
- Ankylosing spondylitis
- Vascular occlusion
- Intrapelvic mass
- Arthritis of hip
- Tumour of ilium or sacrum

All backache is not Disc. Lesion. 12 other important causes must be excluded.

ORTHOPAEDICS AND RHEUMATOLOGY

Lumbosacral Spine
Fig. 97

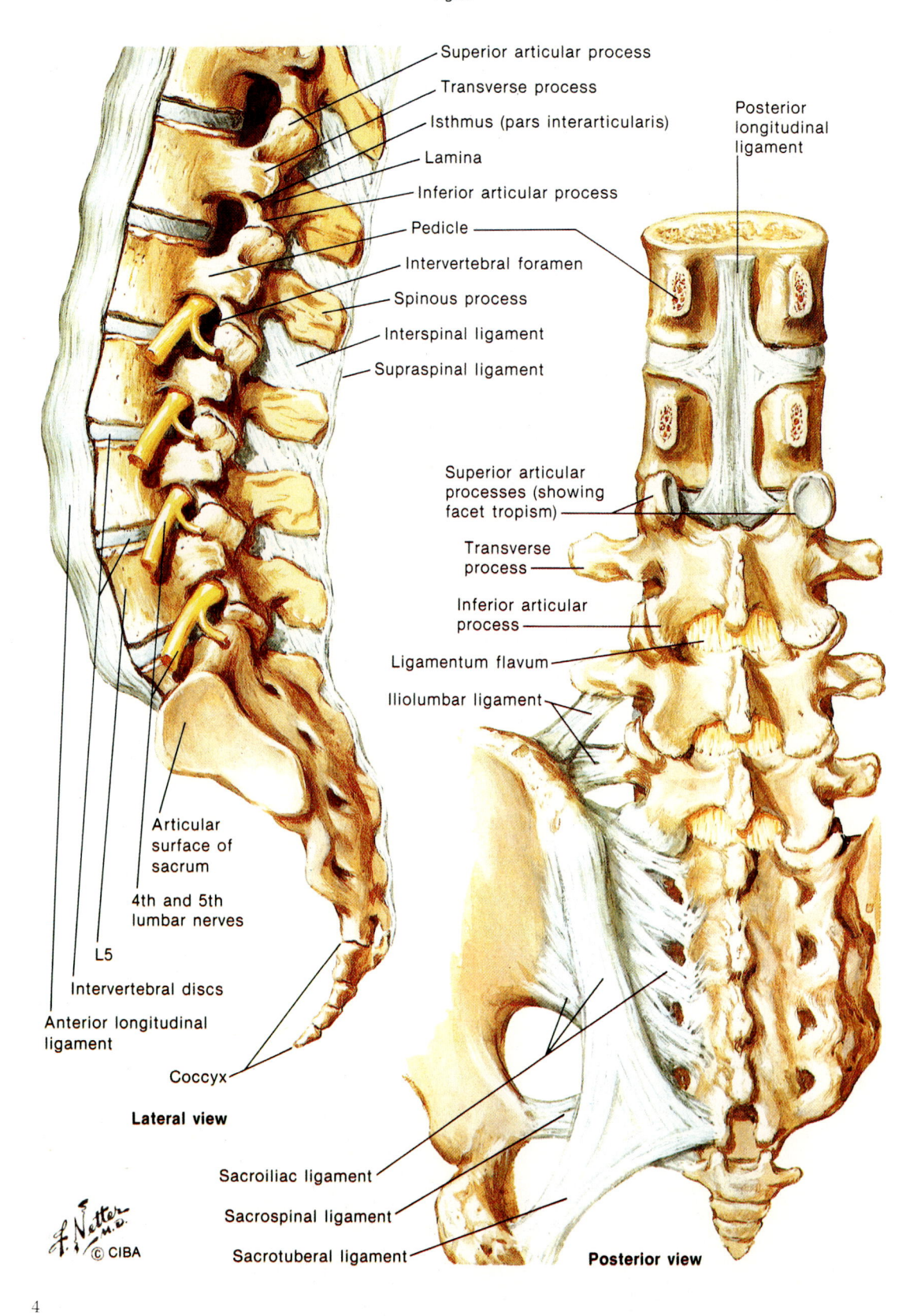

Lateral view

Posterior view

with courtesy and kind permission of Ciba-Geigy Plc, Basle, Switzerland

ORTHOPAEDICS AND RHEUMATOLOGY

Relationship of Spinal Nerves to Vertebrae
Fig. 98

Relationship of Spinal Nerves to Vertebrae

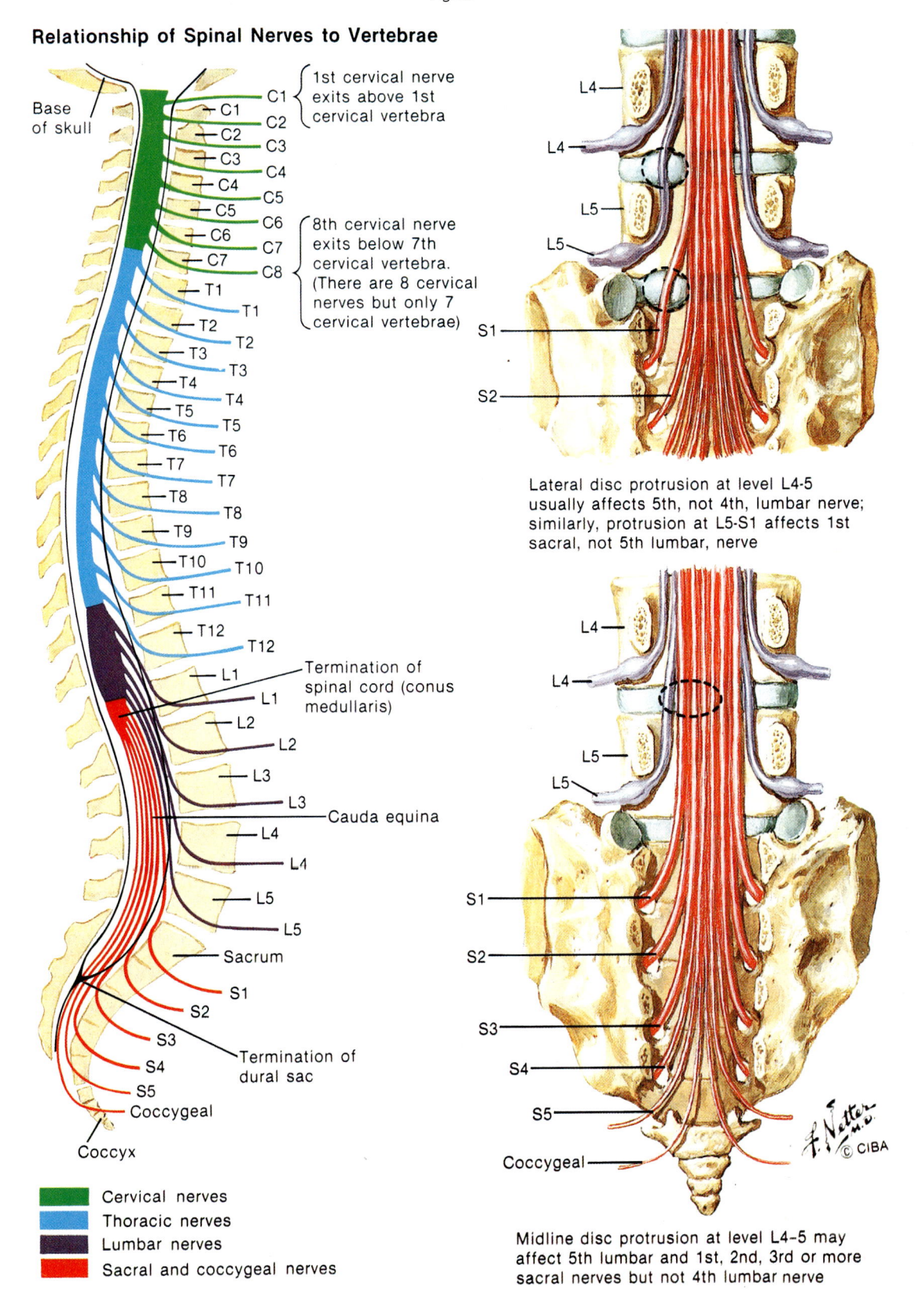

Base of skull

1st cervical nerve exits above 1st cervical vertebra

8th cervical nerve exits below 7th cervical vertebra. (There are 8 cervical nerves but only 7 cervical vertebrae)

Termination of spinal cord (conus medullaris)

Cauda equina

Sacrum

Termination of dural sac

Coccyx

- Cervical nerves
- Thoracic nerves
- Lumbar nerves
- Sacral and coccygeal nerves

Lateral disc protrusion at level L4-5 usually affects 5th, not 4th, lumbar nerve; similarly, protrusion at L5-S1 affects 1st sacral, not 5th lumbar, nerve

Midline disc protrusion at level L4–5 may affect 5th lumbar and 1st, 2nd, 3rd or more sacral nerves but not 4th lumbar nerve

with courtesy and kind permission of Ciba-Geigy Plc, Basle, Switzerland

ORTHOPAEDICS AND RHEUMATOLOGY

Spinal Tumours - Operations

Fig. 99

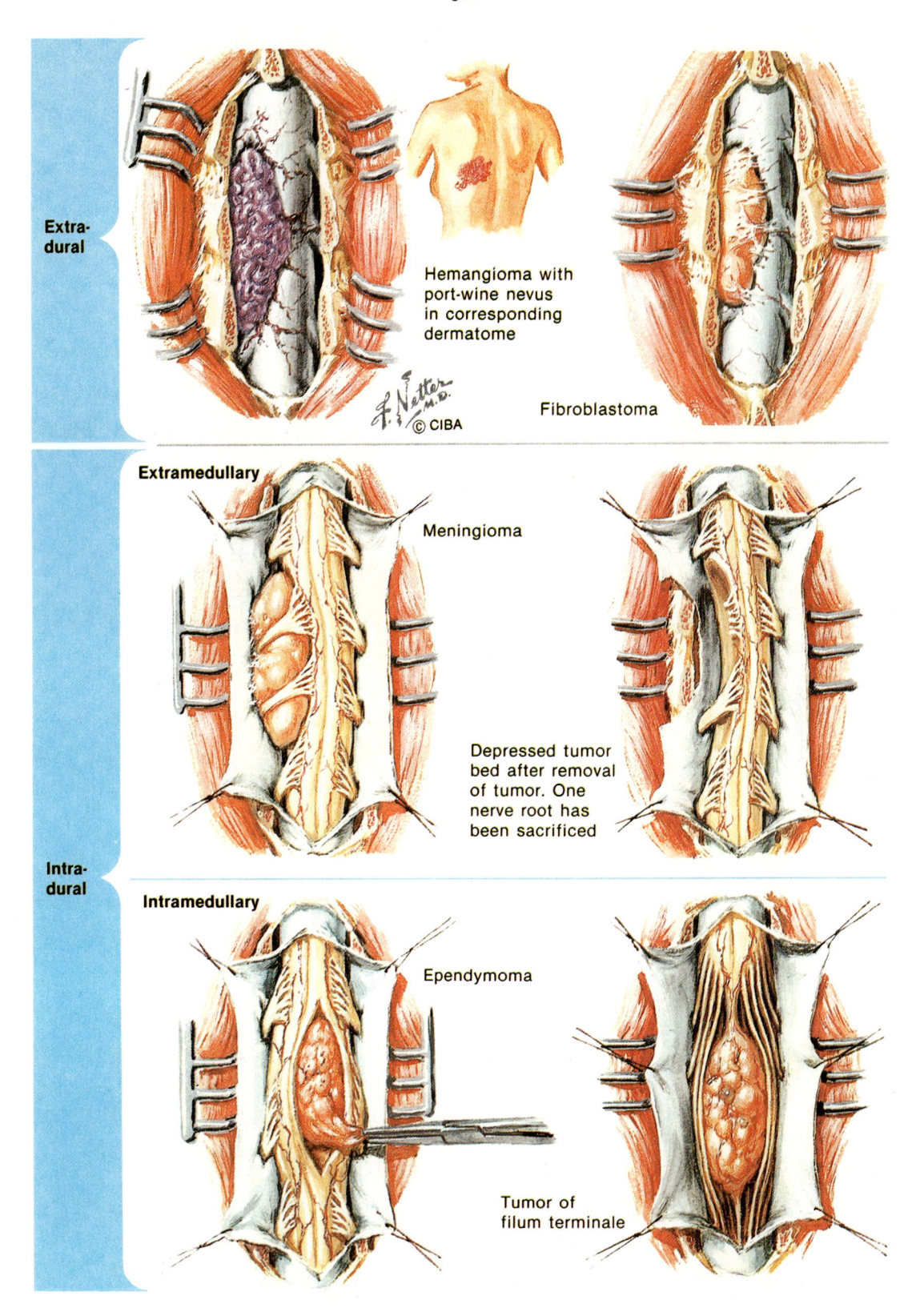

Extradural

Hemangioma with port-wine nevus in corresponding dermatome

Fibroblastoma

Intradural

Extramedullary

Meningioma

Depressed tumor bed after removal of tumor. One nerve root has been sacrificed

Intramedullary

Ependymoma

Tumor of filum terminale

with courtesy and kind permission of Ciba-Geigy Plc, Basle, Switzerland.

ORTHOPAEDICS AND RHEUMATOLOGY

Vertebral Column Tumors

Fig. 100

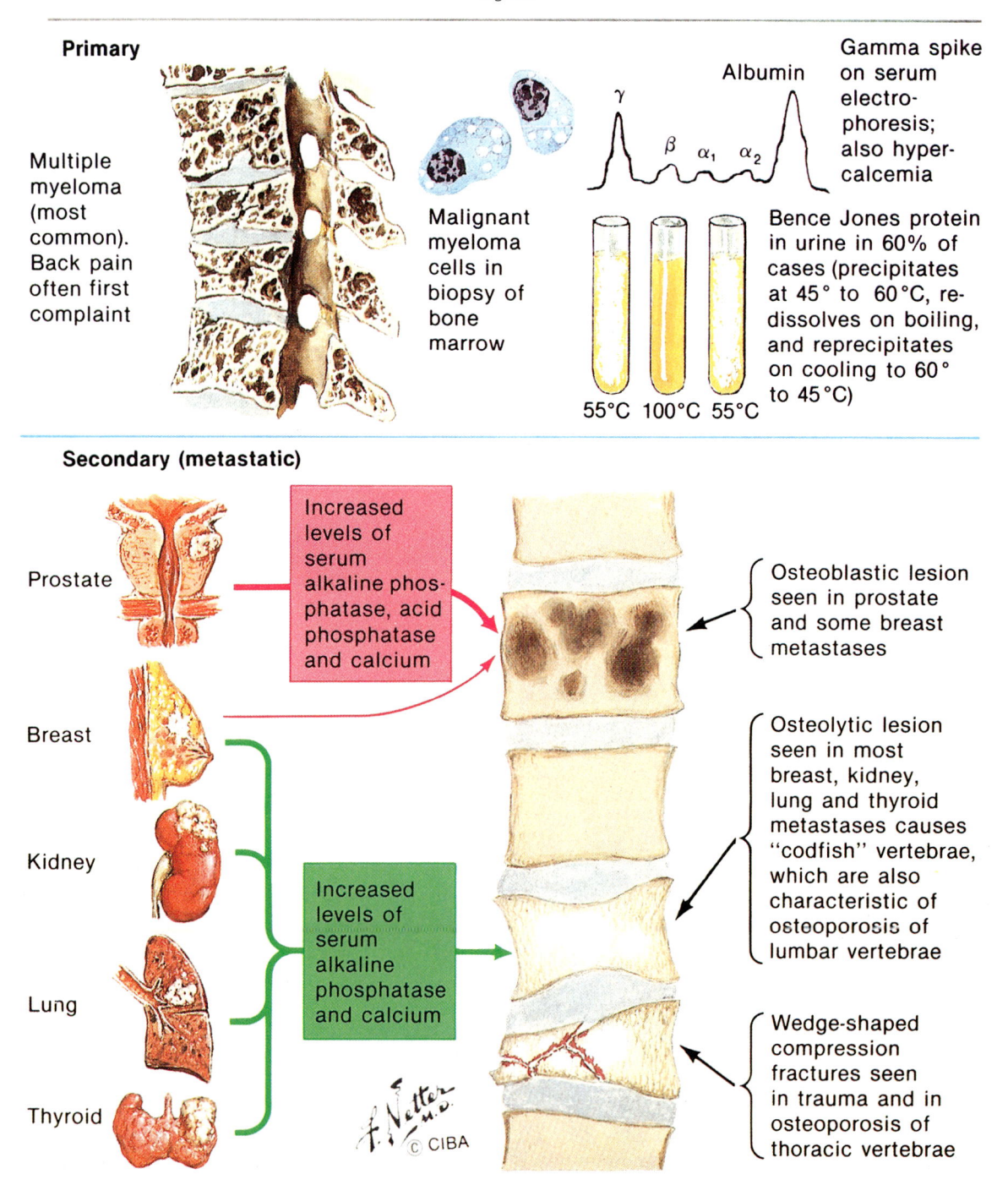

Primary

Multiple myeloma (most common). Back pain often first complaint

Malignant myeloma cells in biopsy of bone marrow

Gamma spike on serum electrophoresis; also hypercalcemia

Bence Jones protein in urine in 60% of cases (precipitates at 45° to 60°C, redissolves on boiling, and reprecipitates on cooling to 60° to 45°C)

55°C   100°C   55°C

Secondary (metastatic)

Prostate — Increased levels of serum alkaline phosphatase, acid phosphatase and calcium → Osteoblastic lesion seen in prostate and some breast metastases

Breast

Kidney

Lung

Thyroid

Increased levels of serum alkaline phosphatase and calcium → Osteolytic lesion seen in most breast, kidney, lung and thyroid metastases causes "codfish" vertebrae, which are also characteristic of osteoporosis of lumbar vertebrae

Wedge-shaped compression fractures seen in trauma and in osteoporosis of thoracic vertebrae

Causes of Primary and Secondary bone tumours of the spine. Investigations must include to find the primary. Secondaries to bone are commonly from bronchus, breast, kidney, thyroid, prostate. Investigations must include X-rays, Ultra-sound, C.A.T. scans. Serum Ca++ (Hypercalcaemia).

with courtesy and kind permission of Ciba-Geigy Plc, Basle, Switzerland

69

ORTHOPAEDICS AND RHEUMATOLOGY

CERVICAL SPONDYLOSIS
(Arthritis of Cervical Spine)

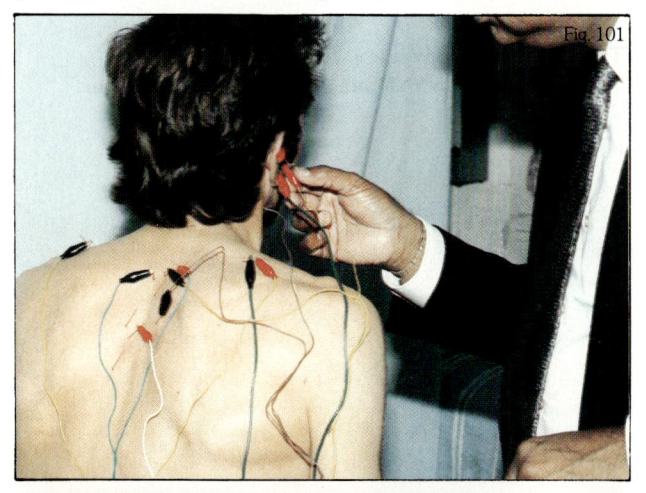

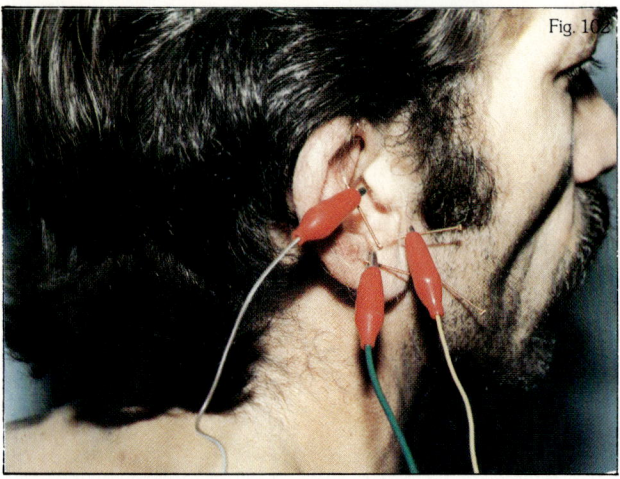

Fig. 101

Fig. 102

Cervical Spondylosis — Lesion C_5 C_6 C_7.
Body Points: Bl_{11} Bl_{13} Bl_{15} GB_{21} GV_{10} GV_{12}.
Ear Points: Cervical Spine. Shenmen. Anti-agression.
Electroacupuncture Bl_{11} GV_{10} GB_{21}. Connect all ear points. Frequency f_1 6 f_2 20 Dense Disperse Current.
Treatment: 20-40 mins. Weekly: 1 Session.

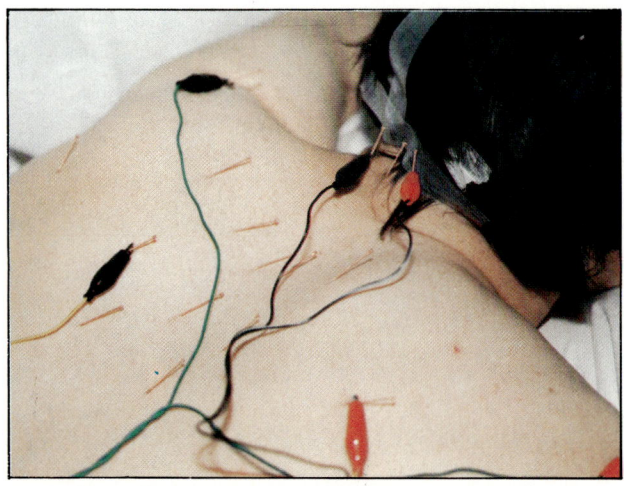

Neck Pain and Inter-scapular Pain
Body Points: BL_{10} Bl_{14} Bl_{17} GB_{21} SI_{11} $GV8$. GV 12, Ahshi points (Tender Pts) needled.
Ear Points: Cervical Spine. Scapular. Shenmen. Anti-aggression. Use both ears.
Electro-acupuncture f_1 6 f_2 20. Treatment 30 mins. Treat once a week.
In all cases ordinary meridians — Bilateral-needling.

LUMBO-SACRAL —
DISC LESION AND SCIATICA

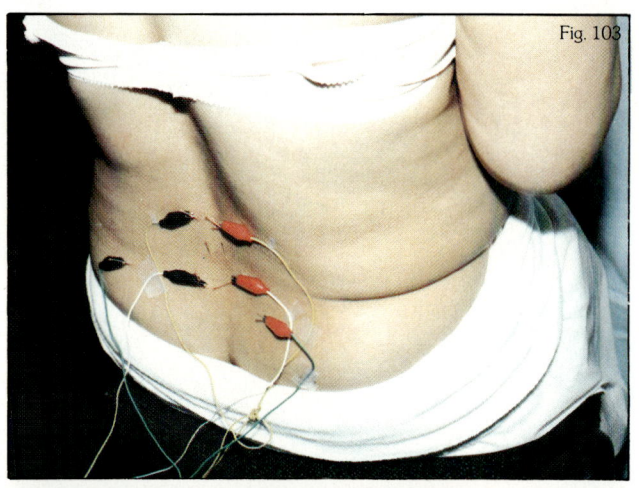

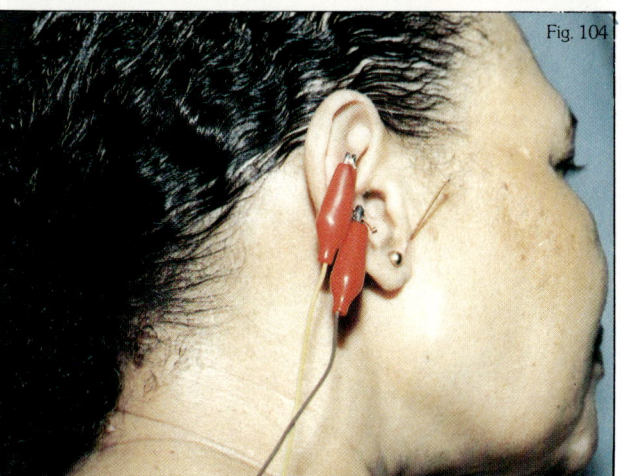

Fig. 103

Fig. 104

Lumbo-Sacral Disc Lesion L_{4-5} S_1
Body Point: Bl_{25} Bl_{27} Bl_{31} Bl_{34} GV_4.
Ear Points: Lumbo-Sacral Spine. Shenmen. Anti-aggression
Electro-acupuncture: f_1 6 f_2 20 Dense Disperse. Treatment: 20-40 minutes each session.
Sessions: Weekly or twice a week.

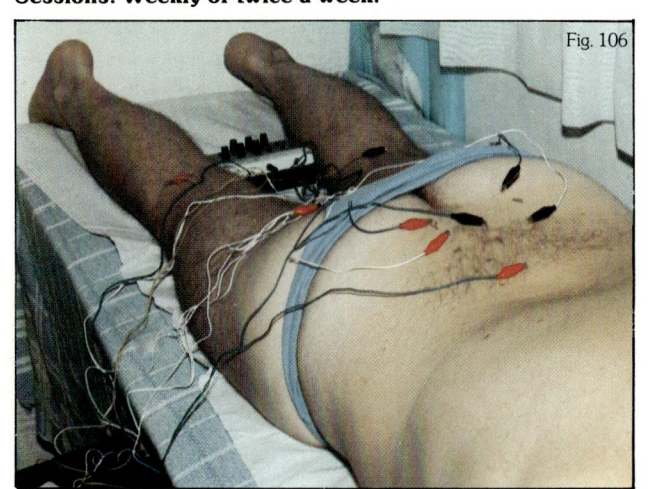

Fig. 106

Burning Pain L_5-Sacrum. Bilat. Sciatica.
Body Points: BL_{31} BL_{34} Bl_{54} (Popliteal Crease) GV_{2-4-6}. Ahshi Point.
Ear Points: L.S. Spine. Lower limb (Triangular Fossa).
Electro-acupuncture f_1 8 f_2 30.
Treat once a week. 4-6 sessions.
Also Ear Points — use both ears.

ORTHOPAEDICS AND RHEUMATOLOGY

RHEUMATOID ARTHRITIS OF BOTH KNEES AND HANDS

Fig. 107

OSTEO-ATHRITIS OF KNEES

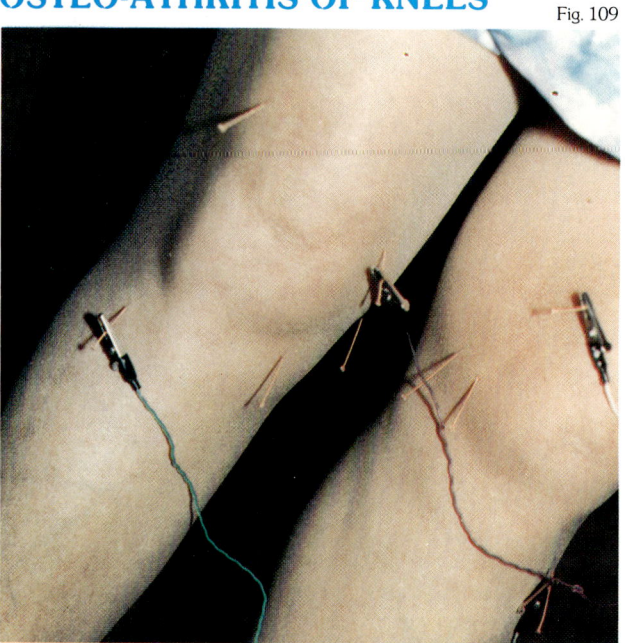

Fig. 109

1. RHEUMATOID AND 2. O.A. OF KNEES

Rheumatoid Arthritis is Auto-Immune.
Osteo-Arthritis is Degenerative.

TREATMENT OF KNEES
Body Points: St_{36} Ki_{10} GB_{34} Sp_6 (Ahshi Pts — Patella)
Ear Points: Triangular Fossa. Anti.Agg. Shenmen.
In Rheumatoid — Thymus Pt level T_2 Ant-Helix as it is Auto-Immune disease

TREATMENT OF HANDS

Body Points. Co_4 $S.I._3$ TH_5.
Ear Points: Scaphoid Fossa.
Electro-Acupuncture f_1 6 f_2 Treatment: 30-45 minutes.
Treatment: Twice Weekly, 10 Sessions.
Thermal therapy with Moxa or Marukyu-Ban Plaster.

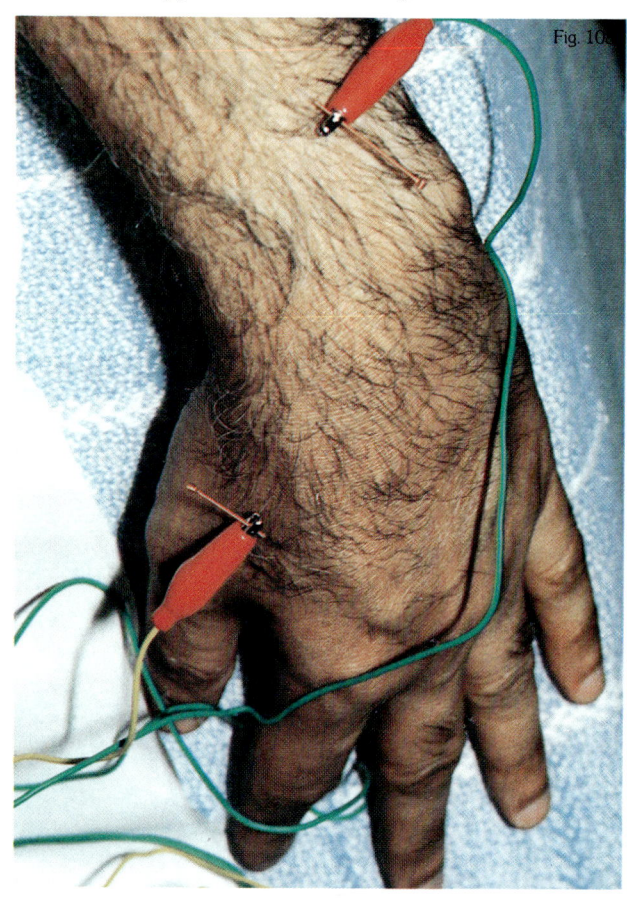

Fig. 108

Arthritis of Wrist and M.P. Joints.
Body Points: CO_4 TH_5 $S.I.3$ Needles at M.P. Joints.

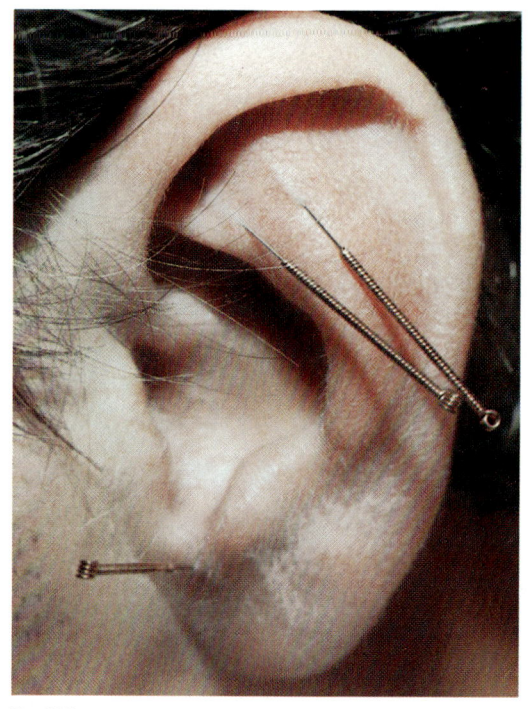

Fig. 110   Ear points used in Arthritis

ORTHOPAEDICS AND RHEUMATOLOGY

Fig. 111

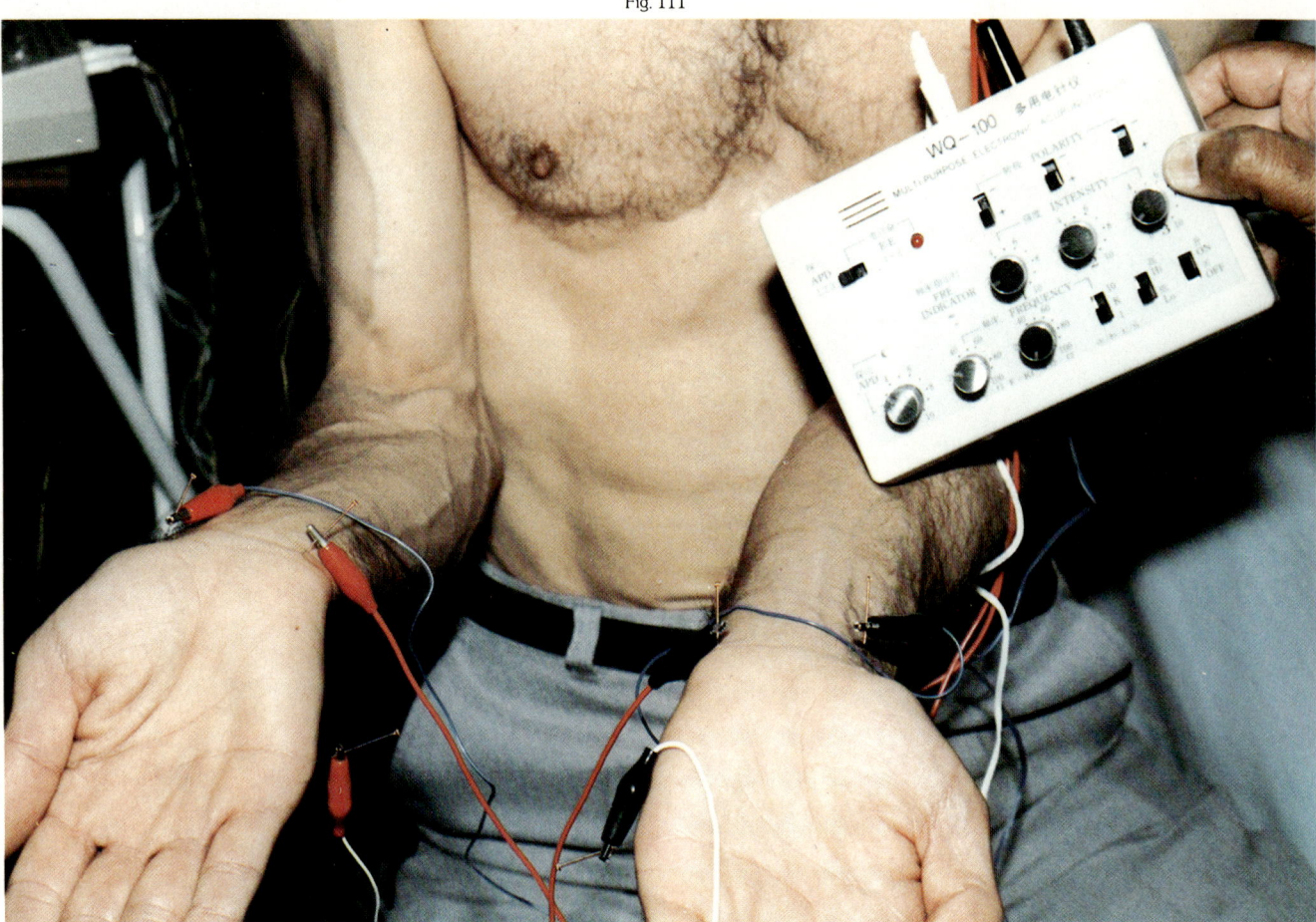

CARPAL TUNNEL SYNDROME
Compression of Median Nerve under Flexor Retinaculum.
9 causes of Carpal Tunnel Syndrome

1. Rheumatoid Arthritis
2. Myxoedema
3. Pregnancy
4. Pill
5. Idiopathic
6. Previous wrist fracture
7. Sarcoidosis
8. Acromegaly
9. Multiple-Myeloma

Numbness or pain and tingling of lateral 3½ fingers.
Body Points: Ht_7 LU_8 SI_3 CO_4
Ear Points: Scaphoid Fossa, Anti-Aggression, Shenmen, Cervical Spine.
Electro-Acupuncture with WQ100 or IC-1107 Acupunctoscope f_1 10 f_2 30 for 30 minutes.
Treatment: Once weekly until symptoms are relieved.

In orthopaedics and Rheumatology Acupuncture treatment is very successful.

It is also used in:

1. Tennis Elbow

2. Golf Elbow

3. Rotator Cuff Syndrome

4. Supraspinatus Tendinitis

5. Ankle Sprain

6. In the treatment of joints like knee, ankle if there is an effusion, the fluid in the joint must be aspirated before acupuncture treatment.

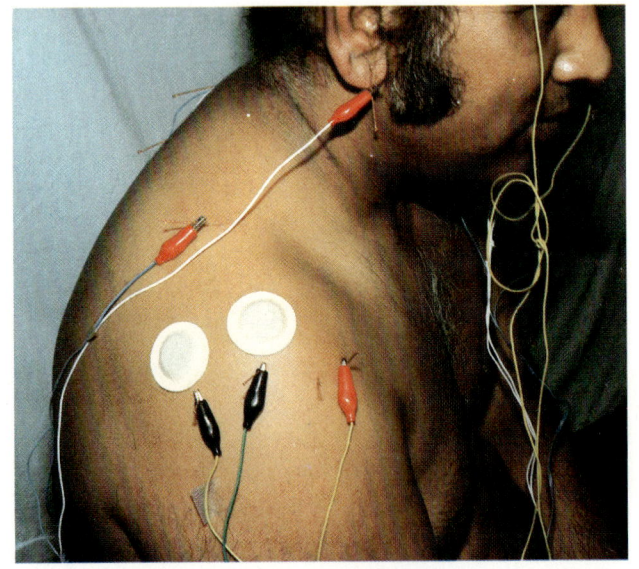

Fig. 112

ARTHRITIS OF SHOULDER
Body Points: CO_4 CO_{11} CO_{15} GB_{21} Ahshi Points.
Ear Points: Scaphoid Fossa. Shenmen. Anti-Aggression.
Electro-Acupuncture: f_1 8 f_2 20 for 40 minutes.
Treatment: Twice a week, six sessions.
Marukyu-Ban or Moxa thermal therapy is essential and important.

Neurology

1. Sensory Pathways from Skin of Face

2. Trigeminal Neuralgia

3. Bell's Palsy

4. Acupuncture Sympathectomy for Peripheral Vascular Disease

5. Meniere's Syndrome or Disease

TRIGEMINAL NEURALGIA

SENSORY PATHWAYS from SKIN of FACE

The Receptors or nerve endings for ORDINARY SKIN SENSATIONS are linked by 3 Neurones with Receiving Centres in the PARIETAL LOBES.

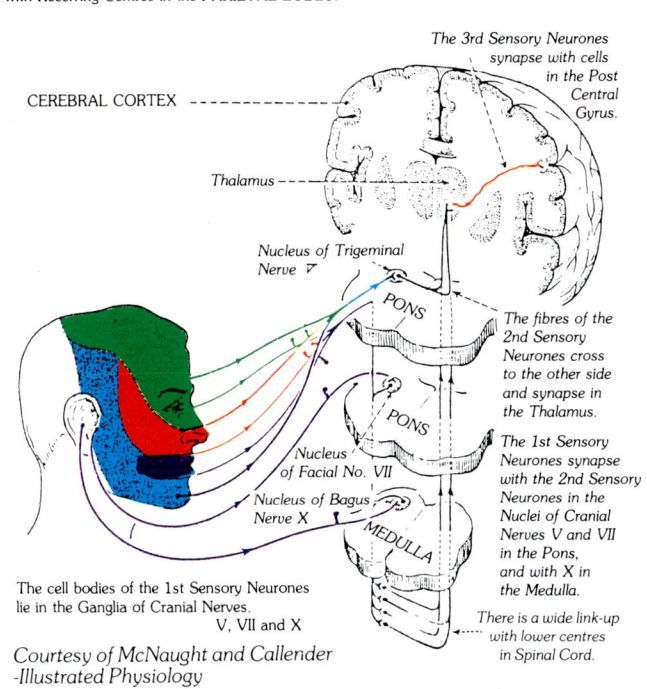

Courtesy of McNaught and Callender - Illustrated Physiology

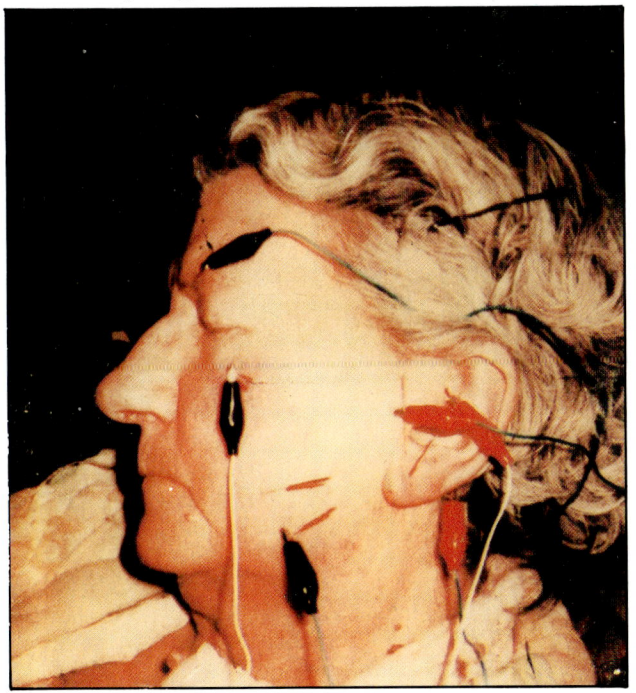

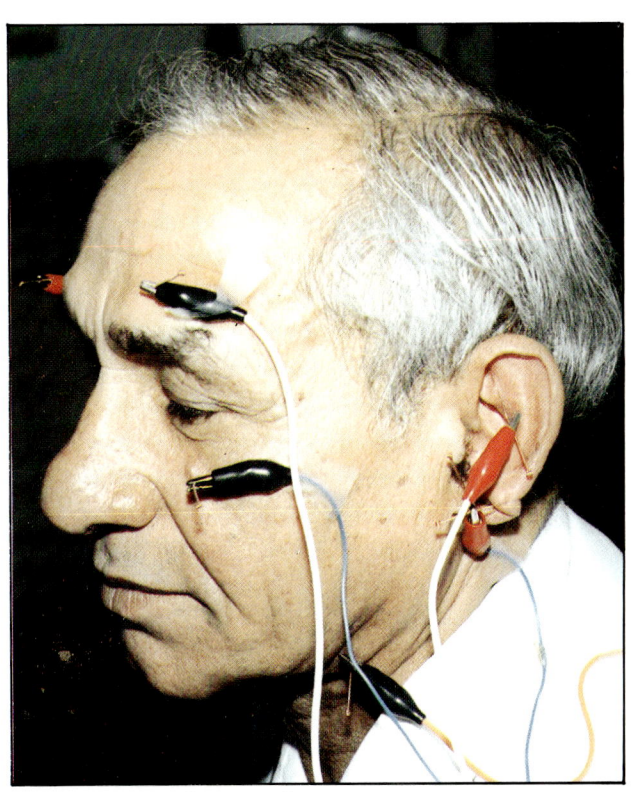

2. Trigeminal Neuralgia

1. Trigeminal Neuralgia

TRIGEMINAL NEURALGIA usually affects elderly Mandibular or maxillary branches usually affected. Ophthalmic occasionally. Trigger factors cold, chewing, touch, shaving etc.

Medical treatment: Slow improvement with Tegretol etc.
Surgery: Ablation of Gasserian Ganglion leaves cornea and side of face anaesthetic permanently - therefore not preferred.
Acupuncture is very successful.
Body Points: GV_{20} CV_{17} TH_{16} CO_4 GB_1 GB_{14} St_2 St_4 St_7 SP_6 St_{36} Li_3
Ear Points: Trigeminal Zone. Thalamus Point, Shenmen, Anti-aggression

Treatment: Electro-Acupuncture 3 times a week. f_1 6 f_2 30. Hertz for 40 mins - at least 1 or 2 sessions weekly, 10 sessions

BELLS PALSY

Fig. 116

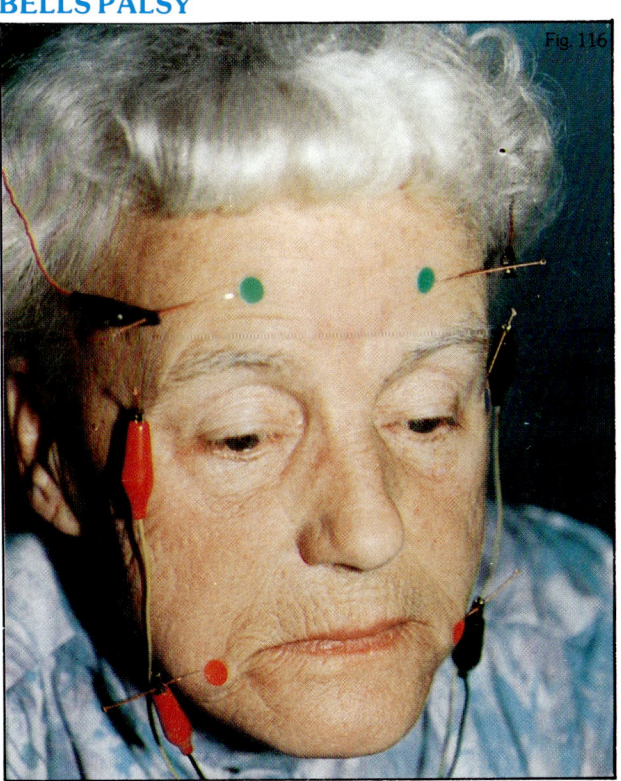

Facial nerve lower motor neurone lesion side of face paralysed. Absence of wrinkling, eyelids can't be closed.
Body Points: GB_1 TH_{23} Bl_2 GB_{14} and St_4.

Ear Points: Facial nerve. Shenmen. Anti-Aggression.

Treatment: Electro-Acupuncture 2 sessions per week - total of 6 sessions. f_1 10 f_2 30 Hertz for 30 - 40 minutes

WQ100 or IC-1107 Acupunctoscope is used.

NEUROLOGY

A. - Acupuncture Sympathectomy for Peripheral Vascular Disease

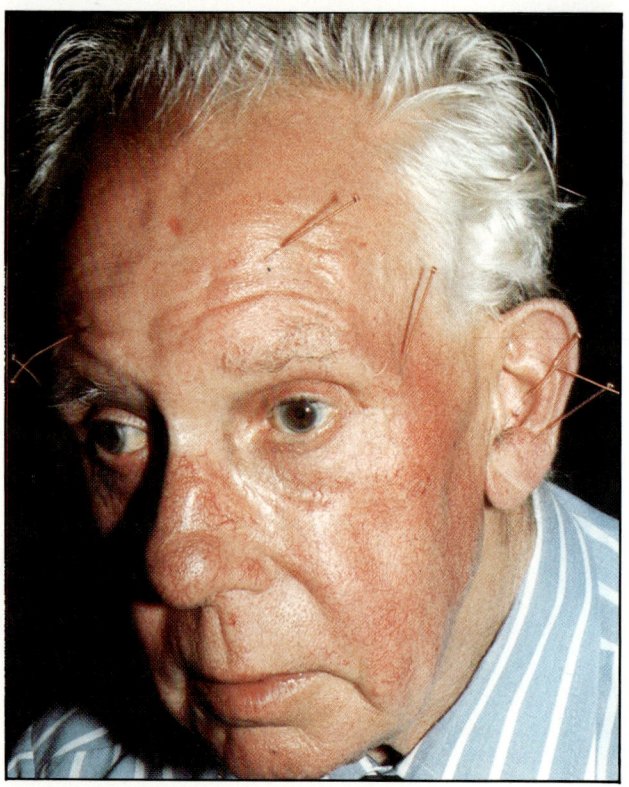

B. - Acupuncture Sympathectomy for Peripheral Vascular Disease
Body Points: Ki_{10} St_{36} Sp_6 St_{41} GB_{43} Bl_{62} St_{41}

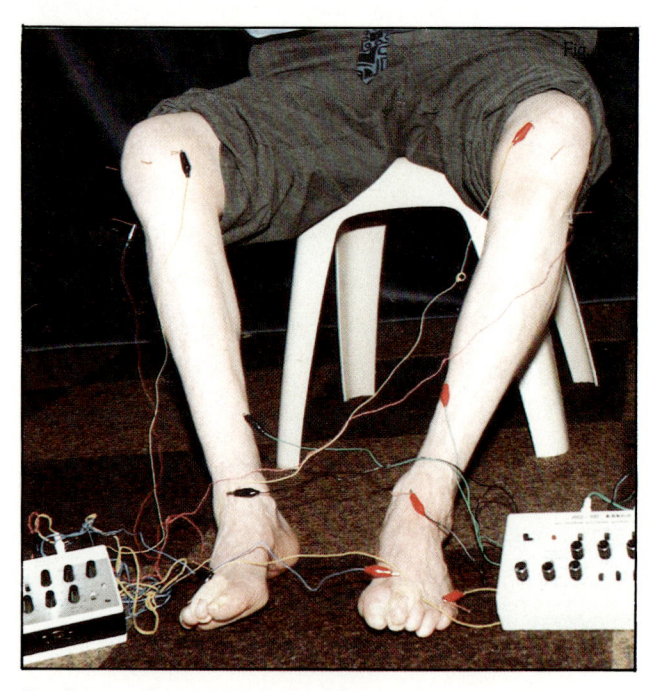

Ear Points: Sympathetic chain inner side of Ant-Helix.
2. Lower limb — Triangular Fossa
3. Shenmen, Anti-Aggression, Hypothalamus
Electro-Acupuncture: f_{10} f_2 40 Hertz.
Stimulate 1 hour.
Treatment: 2 sessions weekly for 10 weeks.

MENIERE'S SYNDROME OR DISEASE
is an affliction of the ear producing dizziness, nausea, deafness.

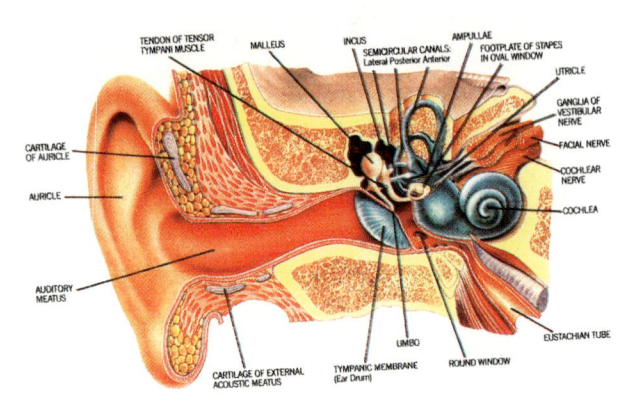

Fig. 119

Meniere's is assocted with fluid endolymph which fills the chambers and canals of the ear known as labyrinth. The cochlea too is filled with endolymph. Due to an increase in the production of endolymph and therefore increase in the pressure of the fluid, deafness, vertigo and tinnitus, occur.

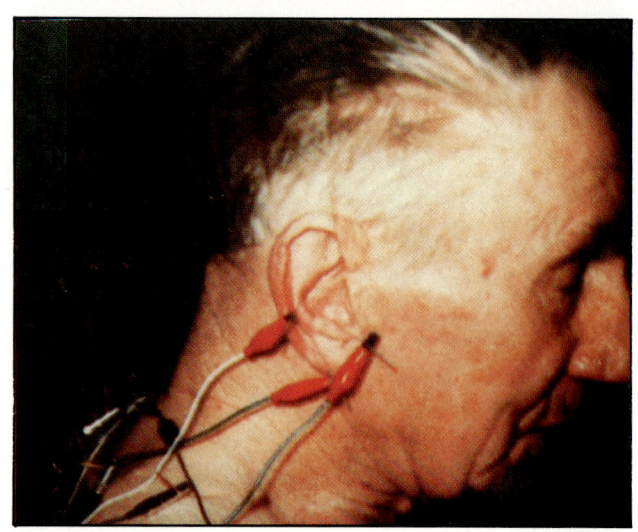

Body Points: GV_{20} CV_{17} TH_{16} GB_{14} CO_4 SI_3 TH_5 Li_3 Sp_6 St_{36}.
Electro-Acupuncture f_1 30 f_2 80 stimulate for 1 hour.
Treatment 3 times each week for 10 weeks.

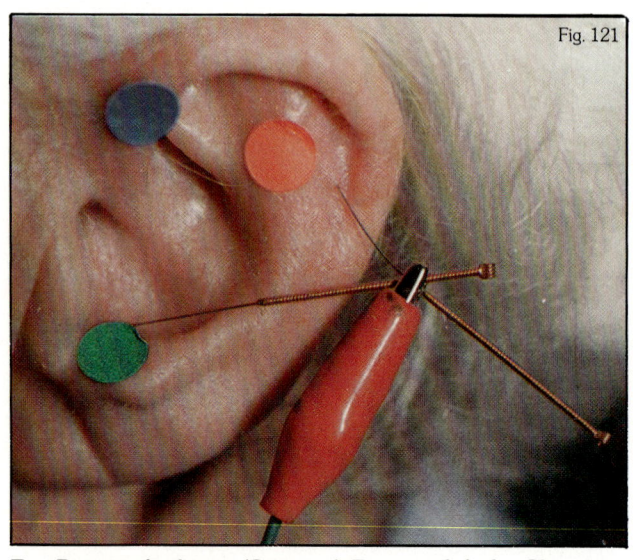

Fig. 121

Ear Points: Auditory (Sensory) Zone in lobule. Shenmen. Anti-Aggression, Internal Ear.

Anti-Smoking and Anti-Obesity Programmes

Anti-Smoking Programme

Four Techniques Available

1. Using Semi-permanent needles only
2. Stimulate and then use semi-permanent needles.
3. Use ear geometry and find points to be used.
4. 10-Needle Technique of Nogier

Anti Obesity Programmes

Four Techniques Available

1. Use Semi-permanent needles only
2. Stimulate and then use semi-permanent needles
3. Use ear geometry and find points to be used
4. In resistent cases or severe obesity, use ear and body points as shown

ANTI-SMOKING

THE ANTI-SMOKING PROGRAMME
FOUR TECHNIQUES

Fig. 122

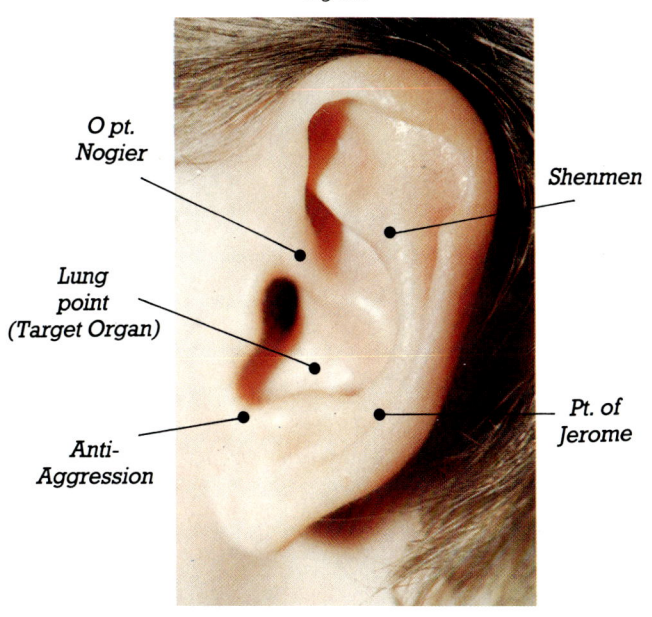

- O pt. Nogier
- Lung point (Target Organ)
- Anti-Aggression
- Shenmen
- Pt. of Jerome

FIRST TECHNIQUE: Use Semi-permanent needles in 1. Lung point. 2. Anti-Agg. 3. Shenman. 4. Jerome.
KEEP NEEDLES FOR 3 WEEKS
SECOND TECHNIQUE: Stimulates above points and then put semi-permanent needles.

Fig. 123

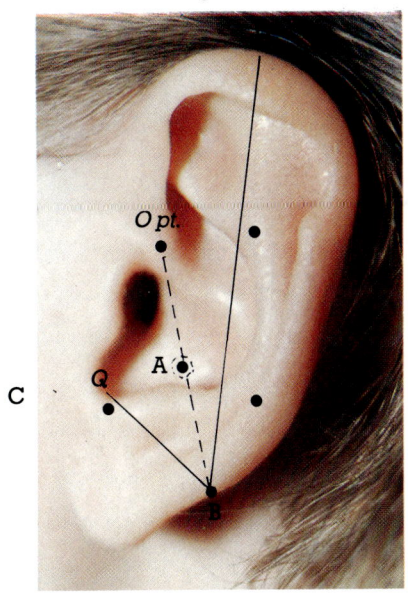

THIRD TECHNIQUE: Using ear geometry. Construct marginal line - join O point to Lung A-B is the marginal line then construct 30° to this line.

Use semi-permanent needles at A. B. C. D. and Anti-Aggression Shenman. Jerome.
KEEP NEEDLES FOR 3 WEEKS

FOURTH TECHNIQUE: Using 10 needles — Nogier 10 needle technique.
5 gold, 4 silver, 1 steel.

Fig. 124

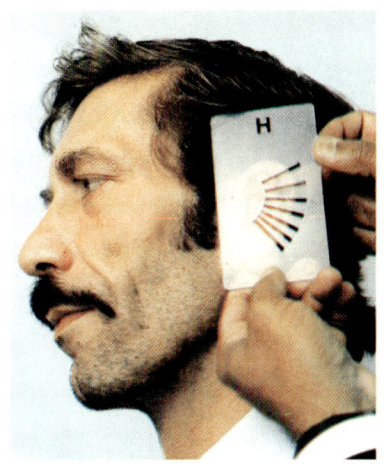

Keep anti-tobacco protractor with highest notch at Darwin's Tubercle. Plastic has 7 slots, 1, 2, 3, 4 slots gold needle, 5th slot — steel, 6th and 7th slots silver needle.

Fig. 125

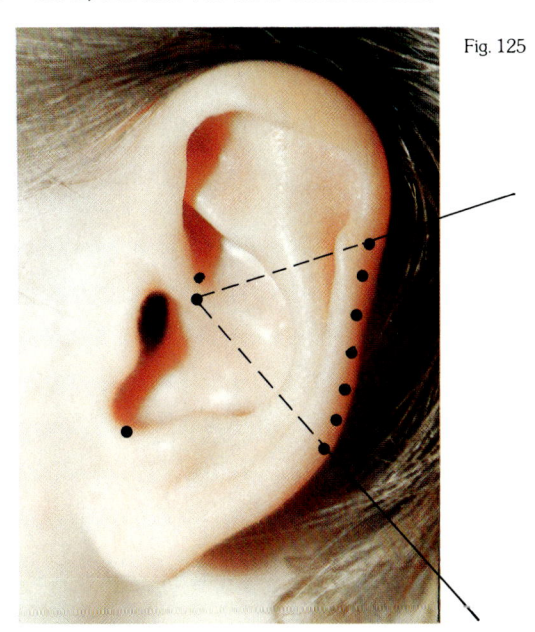

Produced 1st and 7th slot meets at root of Helix. Silver needle at the meeting point, just above this point, insert gold needle. Anti-Aggression - silver needle.
Keep needles for 10-15 minutes and remove.

Fig. 126

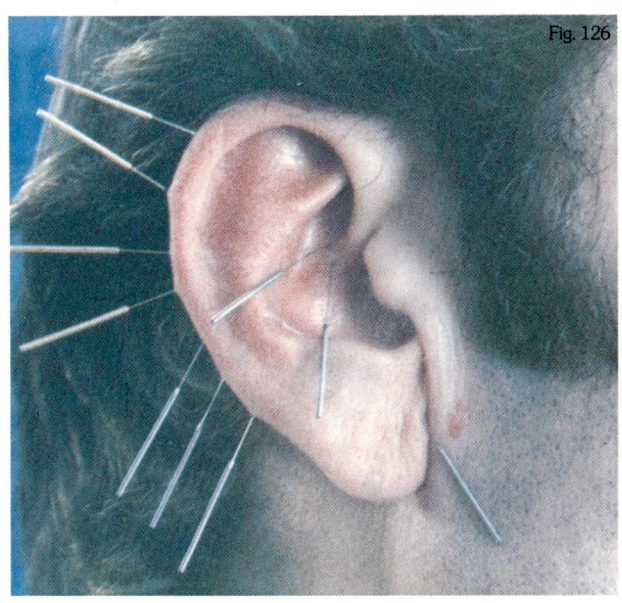

Nogier's 10 needle technique

ANTI-OBESITY

THE ANTI-OBESITY PROGRAMME

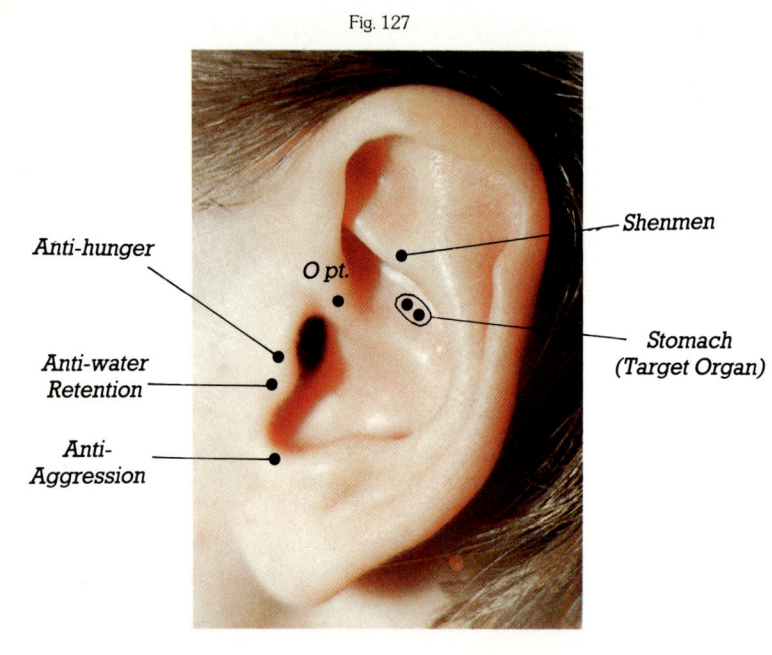

Fig. 127

TECHNIQUE 1: Insert Semi-permanent needles at 1. Stomach. 2. Anti-Aggression. 3. Anti-hunger. 4. Anti-water retention. 5. Shenmen.
Keep needles for 3-4 weeks.

TECHNIQUE 2. Stimulate points and put semi permanent needles.

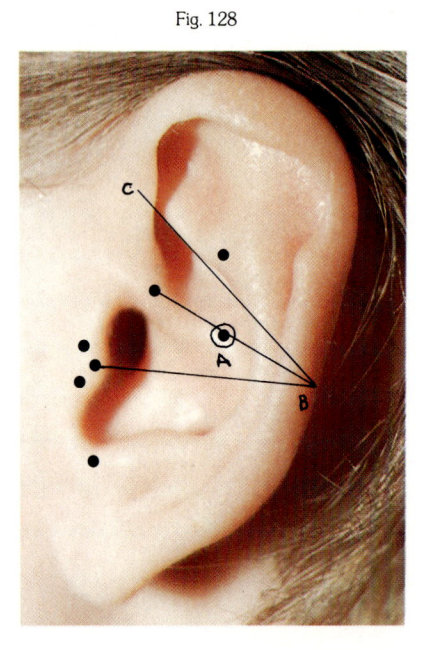

Fig. 128

TECHNIQUE 3. Use ear geometry and put needles at A, B, C, D. Also needles at Anti-Agg. Shenmen. Anti-Hunger. Anti-water. Points on Tragus are Anti-Hunger and Anti-water retention points.

ANTI-OBESITY PROGRAMME IN RESISTANT OR VERY OBESE PATIENTS

In resistant or very obese patients it will be necessary to use ear points as well as Body Acupuncture points and it is essential to use Electro-Acupuncture with the WQ 100 or IC-1107 Electronic Acupunctoscope. Use ear points in all cases.

In resistent or very obese patients use ear and body points.

Fig. 129

EAR POINTS

1. Anti-Hunger
2. Anti water retention
3. Anti-aggression
4. Zero point of Nogier
5. Small Intestine
6. Stomach
7. Shenmen

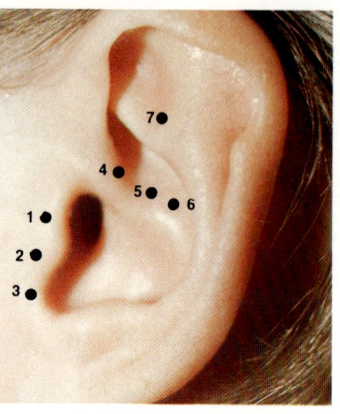

All these above points must be stimulated.
Frequency - $f_1\ 10\ f_2\ 40$
Treatment:— 40 minutes 3 times a week for 4 weeks.
Also body points must be stimulated.

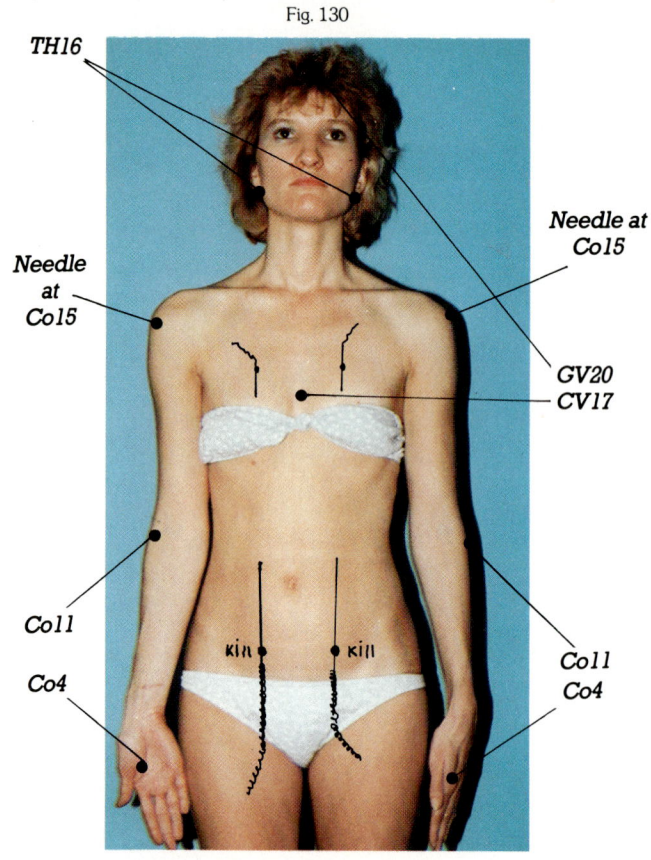

Fig. 130

BODY POINTS

1. Kidney 11 to 22 - 6" needle in kidney meridian. Insert needles as shown ½" lateral to midline.
2. Li 3
3. Spleen 6
4. Co 4

A 6" needle is inserted on either side ½" lateral to the umbilicus from Ki 11 to Ki 22 and stimulated. Other body points are Co_4, Li_3, St_6 bilaterally connected and stimulated.

All points are stimulated - frequency $f_1\ 10\ f_2\ 40$ treat for 40 minutes 2 times a week for 4 weeks.

In very obese patients both ear and body points are essential.

Sinusitis - Headaches

Body and Ear Points

Dermatology

1. Acne
2. Cosmetic Acupuncture for Scars and Wrinkles
3. Insertion of Needle in G.B. 21 - Supra Clavicular Fossa Pneumothorax - Free Method
4. Alopecia
5. Acupuncture Points in Face and Neck for Facial and Neck Pain in general.

HEADACHES

HEADACHES — SINUSITIS

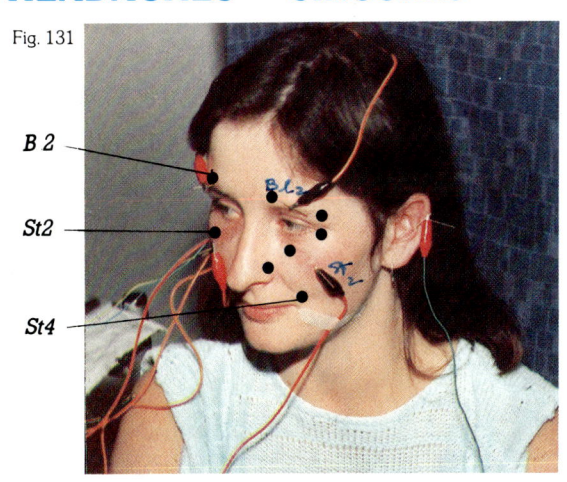

Fig. 131

B 2
St2
St4

Body Points: B_2 $St_{2,3,4}$. GB_1 TH_{23}
Electro-Acupuncture with WQ100 for 30 minutes.

Fig. 132

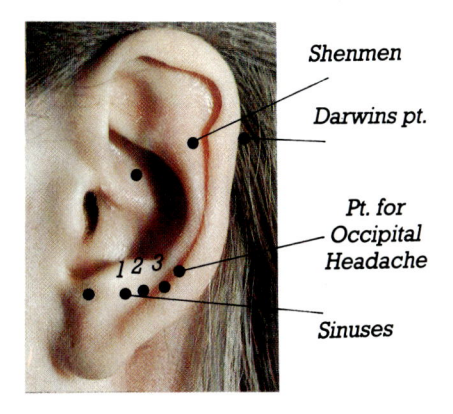

Shenmen
Darwins pt.
Pt. for Occipital Headache
Sinuses

Ear Points: Sinus points and occipital Headache - point in Anti-Tragus.
Anti-Aggression - Darwin's Point.
   Anti Tragus.
Frequency: f_1 8 f_2 30
Treatment: 30 minutes.
One or two treatments.
Insertion of needle G.B.21 in Supra Clavicular Fossa.

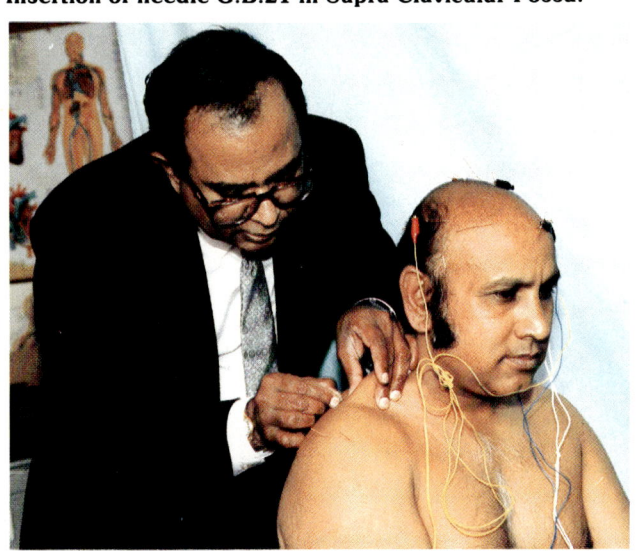

Pneumothorax Free Method. G.B.21 very useful for cervical and shoulder pain. Caution to prevent puncturing Sibsons Fascia. Raise Trapezius and Posterior Muscles of Fossa. Insert needle in an upward direction as shown.

DERMATOLOGY AND COSMETIC ACUPUNCTURE
ACNE

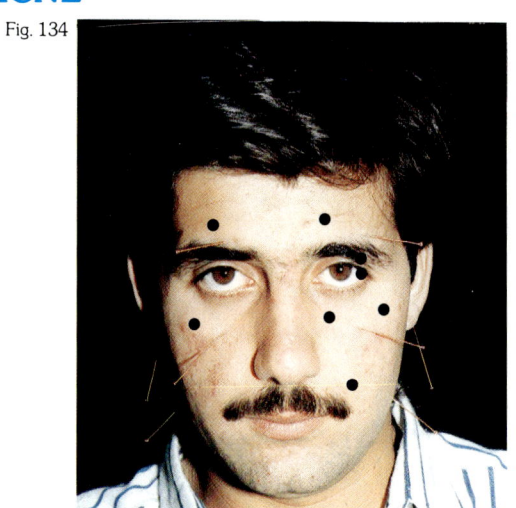

Fig. 134

Acne: Obstruction of sebaceous duct.
Body Points: GB_{14} GB_1 TH_{23} St2, 5
Ear Points: Lobule — Face Area
   Anti-Aggression. Shenmen.

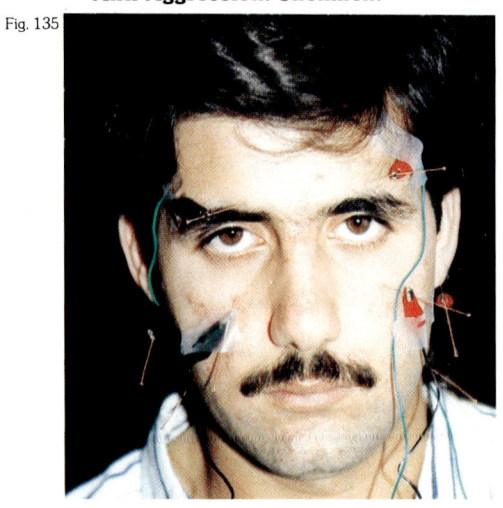

Fig. 135

Electro-Acupuncture WQ100 or IC-1107
f_1 10 F_2 40.
Time: 30-40 minutes.
Treatment: Once a week.

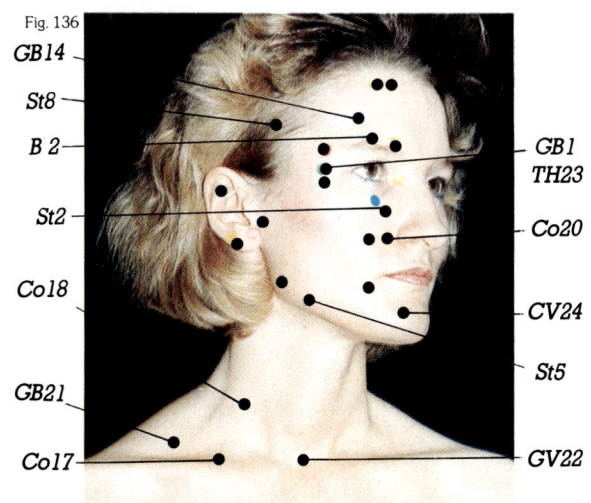

Fig. 136

GB14
St8
B 2
St2
Co18
GB21
Co17

GB1
TH23
Co20
CV24
St5
GV22

Acupuncture points for facial and neck pain in general.

83

COSMETIC — ACUPUNCTURE
ALOPECIA

Fig. 137

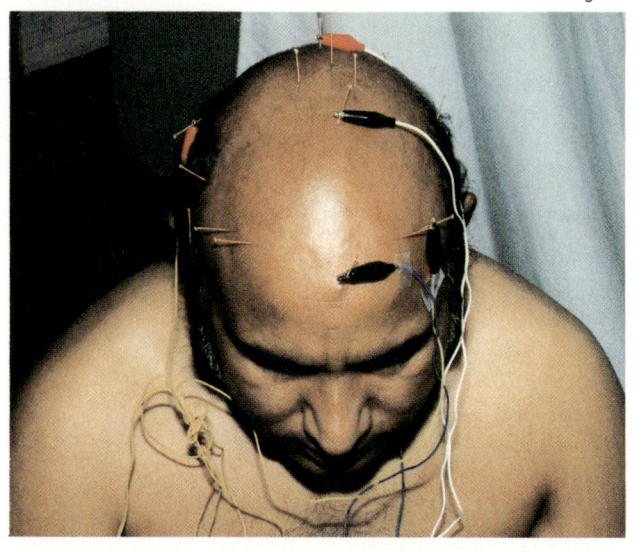

Hair loss in scalp — to the extent till scalp skin is visible is termed Alopecia. Permanent — hair follicles damaged by scarring, e.g. Lichen Planus or Lupus Erythematosus or may recover if hair follicles intact. ALOPECIA AREATA:

1. ALOPECIA AREATA in auto-immune disease: Thyrotoxicosis, Pernicious Anaemia, Addison's Disease. In Down's Syndrome, Vitiligo, Hypo Gamma Globulinaemia.

2. Diffuse hair loss: Hairs lost in Telogen phase, normally 100 hairs are lost per day, endocrine disease. Drugs.

3. MALE PATTERN BALDNESS.
Primary defect is Atrophy of Hair Follicle.
Tt. Body Points: $G.V._{20}$. 4 pt around $G.V._{20}$ GB_{14}. Needle 1" apart like in Corona Technique around Ear Points: Adrenal, A.C.T.H., G.T.H. Scalp area in Lobule. Shenmen. Anti-Aggression.

ACNE AND REMOVAL OF SCARS AND WRINKLES

Fig. 138

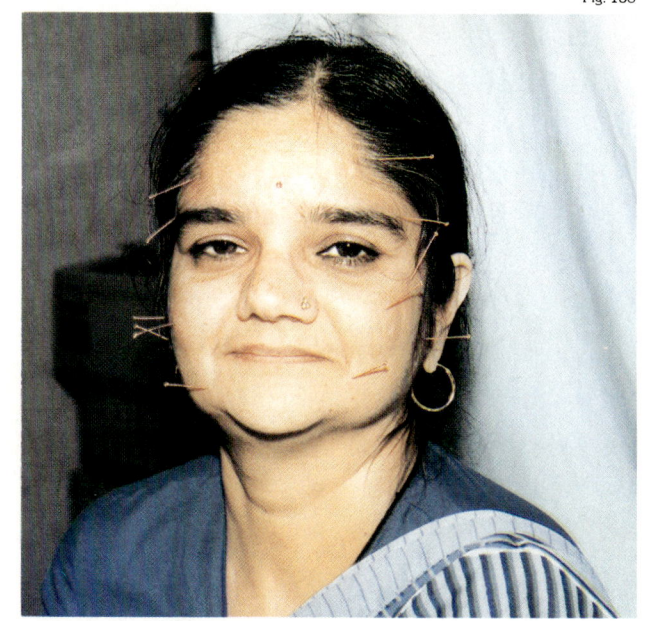

FACIAL — ACNE & WRINKLES
Body Points: Use needles 1" in direction of lines of Langer 6-8 needle each side of face.
Ear Points: Face area in Lobule. Trigeminal zone. Anti-Aggression.
Electro-Acupuncture f_1 20 F_2 100 Daily - 8 sessions.

HEADACHES

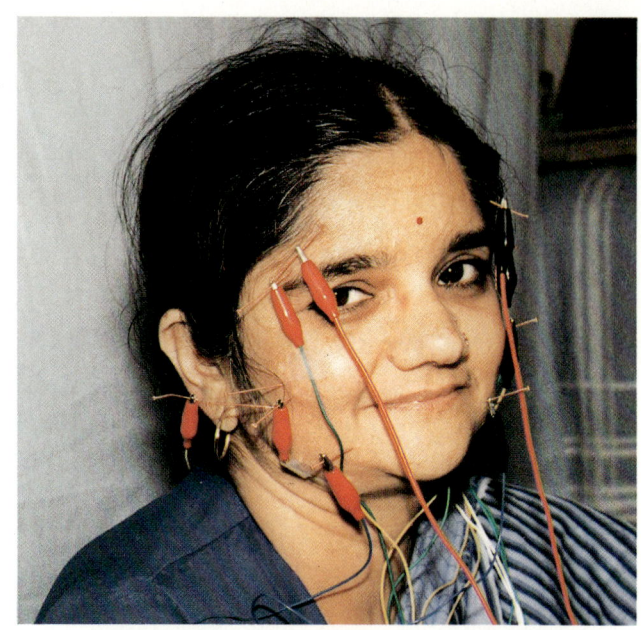

Fig. 139

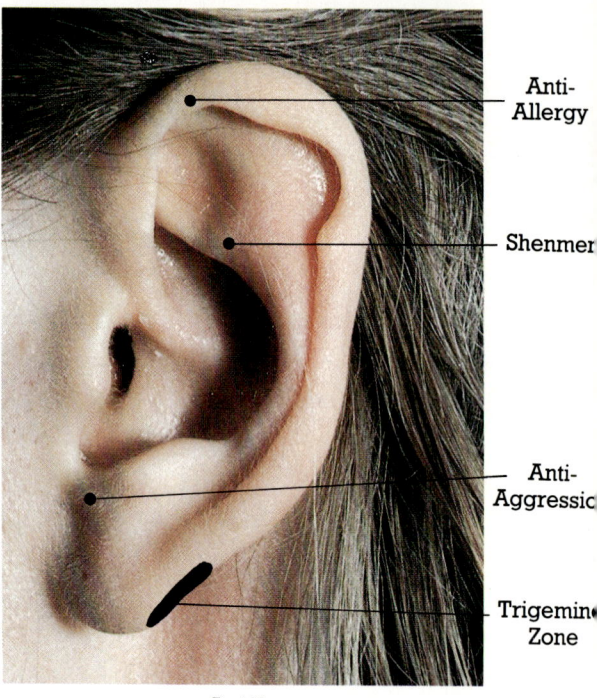

Fig. 140

In using Acupuncture in treating dermatological conditions it is advisable to use both ear and body acupuncture points.

In acne, and eczema etc., there is also an allergic factor and a psycho somatic factor.

Ear Points:—
1. Anti allergy point
2. Anti Aggression point
3. Shenmen points
4. Face point and trigeminal zone shown above - ie. Lobule of Ear.

Body Points:—
Gv20, Cv17, Co4, Co11, Co15, Th16, Sp6, St36, Li3, these are the nervous tension points of the body.

Painless Childbirth

1. General explanation and principles

2. Aim in using Acupuncture in childbirth
    - (a) Mother
    - (b) Child

3. Acupuncture Points used in Painless Childbirth
    - (a) Body Points
    - (b) Ear Points

4. Technique of Electronic Stimulation of Points

5. Electronic stimulation is superior to manual stimulation

6. Contra-Indications - 5 cases unsuitable for Acupuncture

PAINLESS CHILDBIRTH

Birth is a natural event and it is rather an enigma that it should hurt. Pain though is not just a simple response to something unpleasant or harmful, it is highly complex and involves many different mechanisms and pathways.

Old wives tales about the horrors of birth have been dispelled by the proper education given to most parents-to-be today. This trend and the advances of modern medicine have removed many former fears and hazards associated with birth.

Let us take a look at the birth process before we examine the pain associated with it and the specific role acupuncture can play in alleviating this. When a woman learns she is pregnant she usually starts preparation classes which explains the event during the nine months leading up to birth, and teach her relaxation and breathing exercises, so that when the delivery time arrives she is confident and in control.

Doctors recognise three distinct stages in the birth process. The first is the longest and lasts some 8 to 12 hours for a first baby, but may be as short as two to three hours for a woman who has had children before. Sometimes this first stage is induced by injecting the mother with a stimulant that makes the womb contract. Before she is injected, a pessary is inserted into the vagina and the membranes that have enclosed the fluid supporting the baby during its development in the womb are carefully broken, allowing the fluid to escape. If the first stage starts naturally, the membranes break of their own accord, often preceded by a slight blood-stained discharge from the vagina.

The woman's first contractions, whether induced or natural, start as an aching feeling which lasts about 20 seconds and re-occurs every 10 to 20 minutes. By the end of the first stage these contractions last from a minute to a minute-and-a-half at intervals of just three to four minutes. The opening of the womb, the cervix, widens a little more with each contraction in preparation for the baby's passage along the birth canal. The last contractions of this stage, leading to a fully open cervix, are the most painful.

When the cervix is wide open labour has reached stage two. Now the woman can bear down with each contraction, using the exercises taught at ante-natal classes. This stage is typically fairly short, for a first baby it may last 30 to 90 minutes. If it takes longer, or the baby shows signs of oxygen starvation, the delivery can be speeded up by using forceps to ease out the baby's head. Another aid is to make a small slit at the end of birth canal, known as an episiotomy.

Once the baby is delivered, usually head first, the umbilical cord is cut and tied. The third and final stage, lasting 10 to 30 minutes, is the delivery of the afterbirth or placenta.

Some parts of this birth process are painful for the mother and she is commonly offered several alternatives to alleviate her discomfort, including gas and oxygen, painkilling injections like pethidine, lignocaine and trilene, and epidural anaesthesia (injection of an anaesthetic into the lower back). Acupuncture, with the advantages, but none of the drawbacks of these, is an increasingly popular alternative. Its use during labour relieves the pain of contractions and speeds up delivery. In addition, its analgesic effect is useful for manoeuvres like episiotomy, suturing, removal of the placenta and forceps deliveries. The benefits are not only for the mother; the baby suffers no ill effects from the drugs administered to the mother and it less likely to experience oxygen starvation during the contractions.

How does birth using acupuncture differ from a typical birth using Western methods? The difference is not dramatic, its use merely means that far lower doses of birth drugs are needed if any. When it has not happened naturally, the amniotic membranes are ruptured artificially and the mother is generally given a drip; but this is given at a much lower rate than normal because acupucture itself encourages uniform and frequent contractions, which are typically short, this is why the risks of the baby suffocating and the mother being exhausted are reduced.

Five major acupuncture points are used for childbirth (Figure 141). One is on the little toe and is referred to as the specific point of labour; two further points which given an analgesic effect to the lower abdomen and the perineum (genital area) are on the outside of the mid-calf and just above the ankle; and the remaining two are on the hand and on top of the head. The point on the head is needled first, and the remaining needles are inserted on the woman's left side so that the midwife or obstetrician is free to work on the right side when birth is imminent (during the second stage). Delivery time can be reduced even more if the hand and little toe needles are inserted on both sides of the body, but this is not essential.

Once in position, the needles are stimulated to induce the painkilling effect. The one in the hand is best manipulated manually by the doctor to coincide with the onset of each contraction. Meanwhile, the two leg points are stimulated electrically, using an acupunctoscope. A dense-disperse type current of fairly high frequency (approximately 100 Hertz) is used at an intensity of just five to nine volts (for a full explanation of electro-acupuncture refer to Section 3). The doctor initially sets the machine to deliver a very low frequency stimulation. He increases the frequency gradually until the woman feels the pains of labour masked by a sensation of numbness. This feeling, often described by others as a heaviness or distension, is due to the action of the body's natural painkillers which are released by the acupuncture. Occasionally the relief is inadequate and in such cases small doses of painkilling drugs, local anaesthesia or gas are given to supplement the acupuncture.

The aim in using acupuncture in childbirth is: to the mother:

1. Relieve pain of childbirth.
2. Utilise the analgesic effect of acupuncture for manoeuvres such as:
   a. Episiotomy
   b. Suturing
   c. Removal of placenta
   d. Forceps deliveries

To the child:

To deliver a child with the best chance of survival with least toxic effects of drugs and to relieve hypoxia during contractions.

PAINLESS CHILDBIRTH

ACUPUNCTURE POINTS USED

Body Points:
1. G.V. 20.
2. Bladder 67 (specific point of labour) Bilateral.
3. Spleen 6.
4. Extra point midway between knee and ankle joints.
5. Colon 4. All bilateraly connected.

Ear points:
1. Uterus.
2. Shenmen.
3. G.T. point.
4. Anti-Aggression point.
5. Jerome point: Connect both ears to simultaneous point i.e. to the uterus, shenmen and anti-agression points.

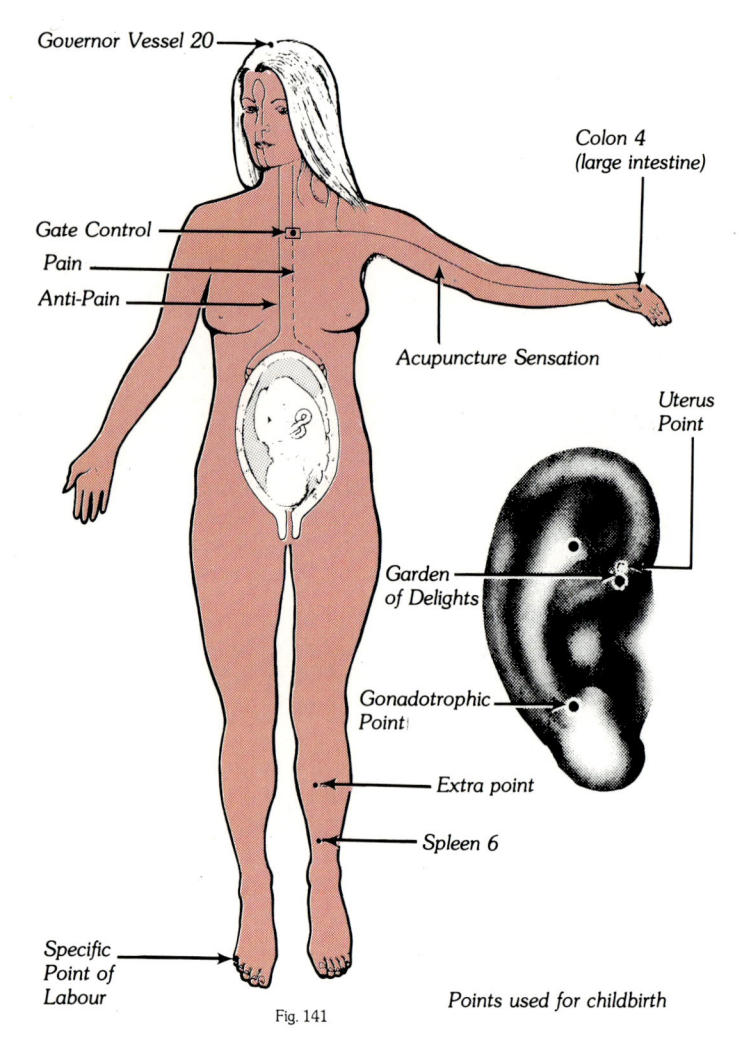

Fig. 141 — Points used for childbirth

Labels on figure: Governor Vessel 20, Gate Control, Pain, Anti-Pain, Colon 4 (large intestine), Acupuncture Sensation, Uterus Point, Garden of Delights, Gonadotrophic Point, Extra point, Spleen 6, Specific Point of Labour

TECHNIQUE AND ELECTRONIC STIMULATION OF POINTS

As contractions start — insert needle at G.V.20 then CO_4 Bl_{67} Sp_6 and Extra point.

Connect Bl_{67} to Bl_{67} Co_4 to Co_4 Extra point and Sp_6 with WQ100 electro-acupunctoscope. Stimulated as follows:

The two needles in the leg u.Ex. and Sp.6 are connected to the pulse stimulator.

Frequency of pulse adjusted to 100 Hertz. $f_1 O_1 f_2 100$ Intermittent Dense-Disperse current.

Intensity — 5-9 volts.

Current — pulsatile current of dense-disperse type is used.

Intensities of stimulation is gradually increased depending on patient's sensitivity and tolerance to the stimulator until the patient felt a sensation of:-

Numbness, soreness, heaviness and distention which masks the so-called 'pains' of labour.

Amniotomy (A.R.M.) is done immediately following stimulation of Co.4.

Syntocynon infusion is started following A.R.M.

Stimulation with WQ100 acupunctoscope should be throughout all stages of labour:
Stage 1, 2 and 3.

MANUAL STIMULATION

This method can be used in the management of painless childbirth but it is not superior to electronic stimulation. The points used are the same but it is uncomfortable to the patient and cumbersome to the doctor.

In painless childbirth if the mother has other medical conditions this must be treated with conventional methods.

Syntocynon infusion can be used but smaller doses will be necessary.

CONTRA-INDICATIONS

1. Cephalo - Pelvic disproportion
2. Placenta praevia
3. Diabetes complicating pregnancy
4. Cardiac disease complicating pregnancy
5. Pre-eclamptic toxamia

The value of needling for relieving birth pain was analysed statistically by Wilfred Pereira, F.R.C.S.(Eng.), F.R.C.S. (Edin.), F.R.C.O.G., President of the Acupuncture Association of Sri Lanka, in 1977. He recorded 110 births that involved the use of acupuncture and divided its success into four grades, based on the degree of pain felt by the mother and the need to use drugs like pethidine, lignocaine and trilene.

In 90 per cent of Pereira's women, with acupuncture there was excellent releif of pain and the mother was calm and needed no drugs. He also counted cases where there was fair analgesic effect, but the mother felt pain at certain stages (small doses of lignocaine were given to these women).

In only 10 per cent of his women was acupuncture classified as 'ineffective'. For these there was either incomplete pain relief, requiring moderate doses of the painkiller pethidine and local anaesthetic, or there was marked pain and acupuncture was discontinued.

Pereira's results confirmed that the majority of women can give birth without drugs when acupuncture is used. They also showed a lower incidence of forceps deliveries than in drug-assisted births.

How can acupuncture relieve childbirth pain? Though the full answer is not yet known, three factors are definitely involved. Before looking at these we must analyse the nature of pain.

When pain is perceived many complex mechanisms and pathways come into play. Nerve fibres at the pain source, in this case the lower abdomen, transmit pulses of information to the brain at speeds determined by the thickness of the individual fibre. Large fibres conduct impulses at a faster rate than small fibres and the outcome of this is that the pulses of information to the brain at speeds determined by the thickness of the individual fibre. Large fibres conduct impulses at a faster rate than small fibres and the outcome of this is that the pulses of information reach the brain in a pattern of impulses that are separated both by space, amongst the different nerve fibres, and time. The brain's interpretation of these patterns depend on its assessment of their significance and where they come from.

PAINLESS CHILDBIRTH

Fig. 142 **Body Points**
- GV20
- Extra Pt.
- Sp6
- Bl 67 — Specific Pt. of Labour

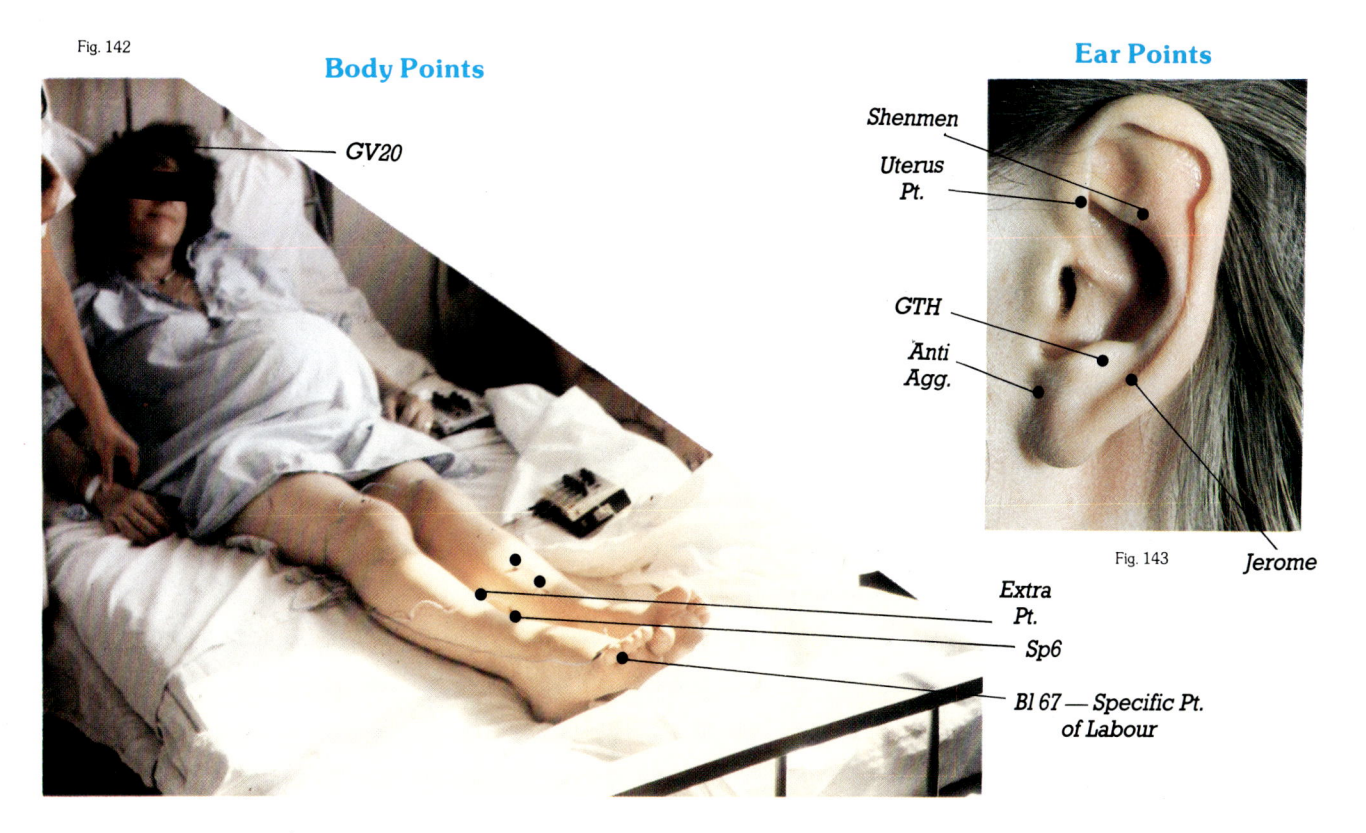

Ear Points
- Shenmen
- Uterus Pt.
- GTH
- Anti Agg.
- Jerome

Fig. 143

Fig. 144 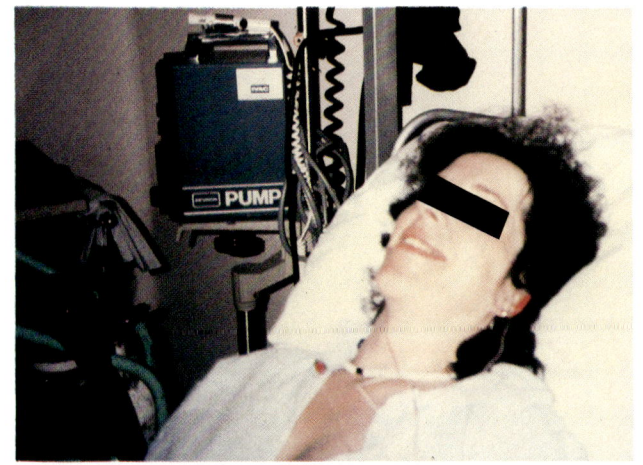
Ear Points connections — First Stage.

Fig. 145 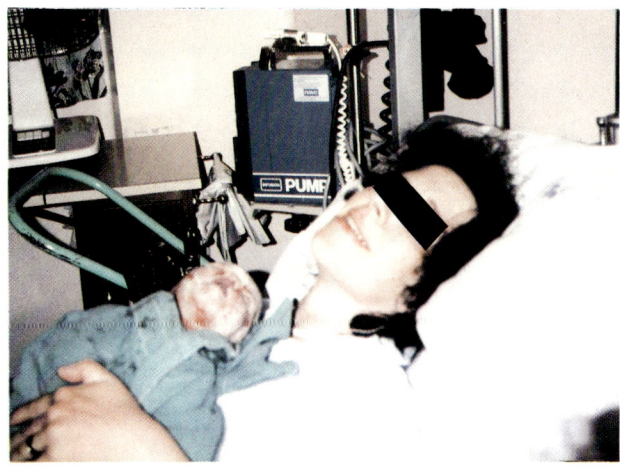
Baby born - mother felt no pain during labour. Stage 1 to Stage 3 lasted 4 hours 40 minutes.

Fig. 146 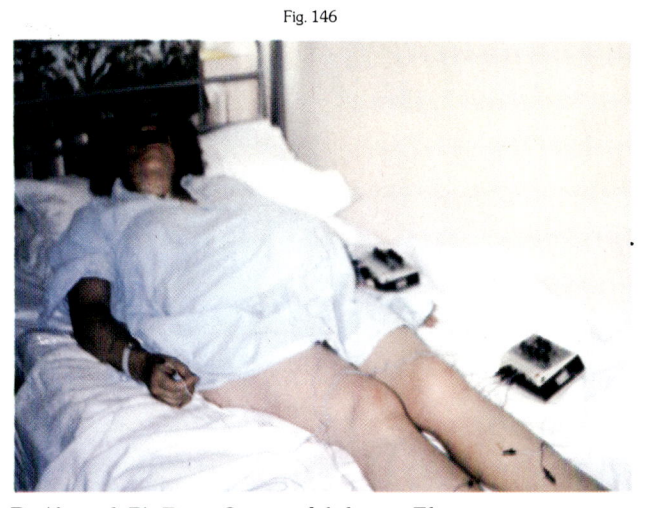
B. (A and B) First Stage of labour. Electro-acupuncture with two WQ100 machines. Frequency f, 0 - f$_2$ 100 intermittent dense-disperse current.

Fig. 147 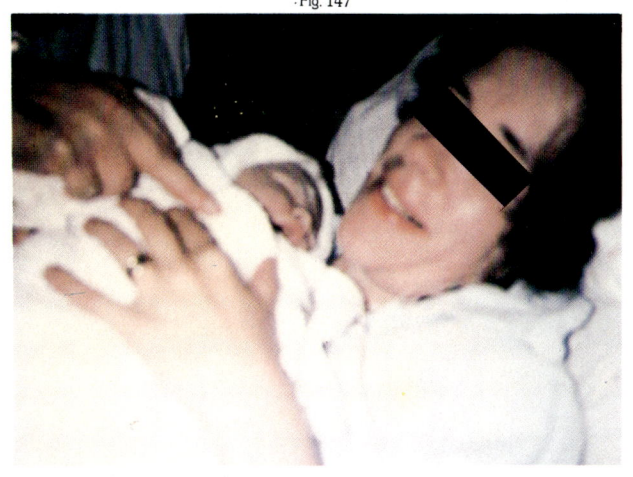
Mother holding baby few minutes after delivery. Remove all needles 5 minues after delivery of placenta.

89

Psycho-Somatics

1. Nervous Tension Points

2. Anxiety

3. Phobias

4. Depression

PSYCHO - SOMATICS

PSYCHOSOMATICS or NERVOUS TENSION POINTS (NTs) OF THE BODY AND EAR

It is widely accepted that every illness has its psychosomatic element. Based on this assumption, the points for nervous tension are generally used in addition to the points specific to the ailment. These nine points, often called NTs are shown in Figure 148 and 149. All are located on the body meridians. They are Liver 3, Spleen 6, Stomach 36, Colon 4, 11 and 15, Three Heater 16, Conception Vessel 17 and Governor Vessel 20.

Whatever the complaint, it is important that an adequate amount of time be allocated to each session of treatment. The first one may take 30 to 40 minutes and if subsequent sessions are necessary these will last at least 15 to 20 minutes each. It is a complete waste of time to treat the patient for just five minutes, because at least 10 minutes of stimulation are needed to induce the release of the body's biochemicals like the neurochemical transmitters, endorphin and encephalin (natural opiates), and hydrocortisone etc.

The number of sessions required varies, sometimes one is enough, on average six to eight are required and in long standing chronic diseases anything from 12 to 20 are necessary. Some conditions just require booster sessions every three to four months. The time between sessions for the average therapy length of six to eight sessions should be no more than a week and sooner if practical.

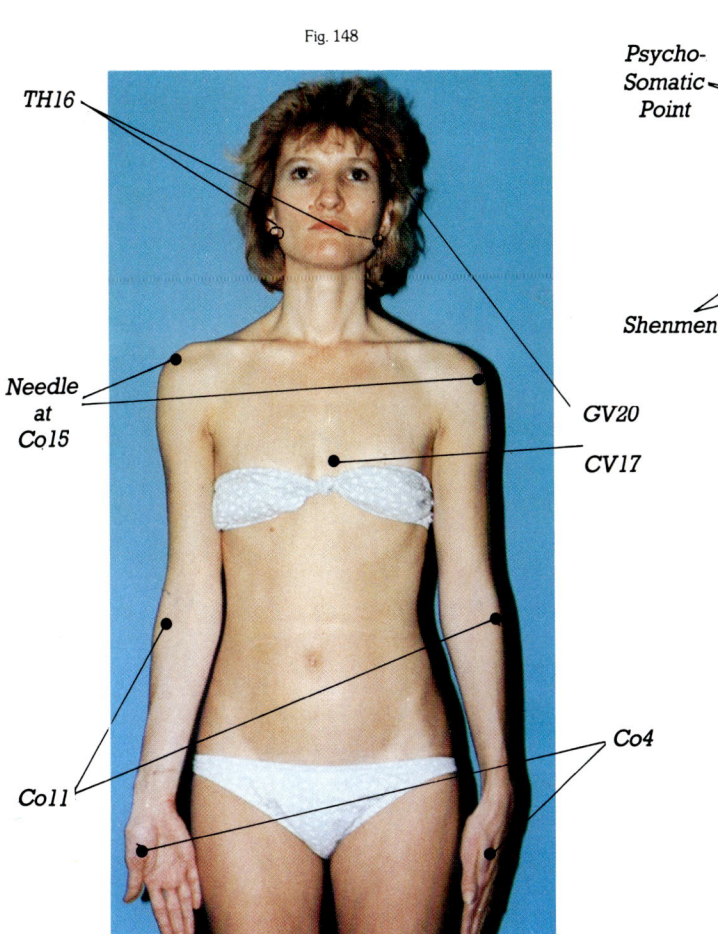

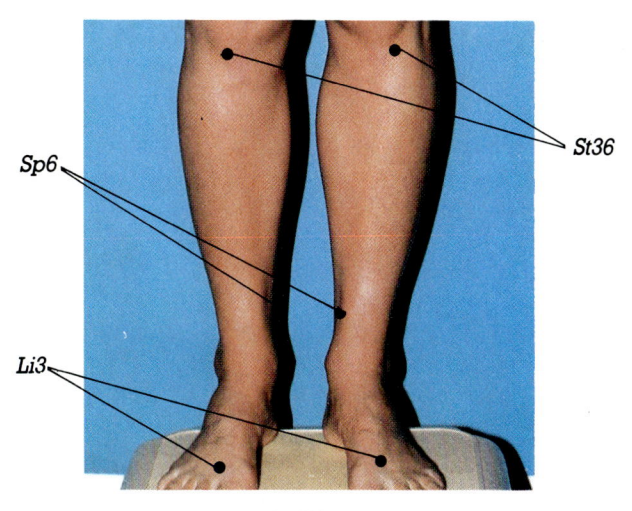

Fig. 148

Fig. 149

These points which are referred to as NTs for short can be used for:
1. Anxiety 2. Depression 3. Phobias 4. Tension etc.

Body Points: G.V.20, C.V.17 — single
Bilateral CO_4 CO_{11} CO_{15} TH_{16} in upper limb
Li_3 Sp_6 St_{36} in lower limb

Ear Points:
1. Anti-Aggression (Cribriform needling will be required if severe tension).
2. Shenmen.
3. Darwin's Point.
4. Pt. De Jerome.
5. Psychosomatic point.

All points and connection with WQ100 Acupunctoscope will be shown below.

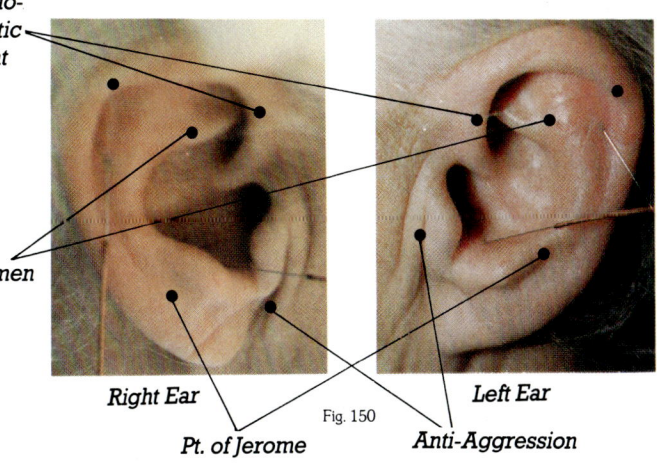

Fig. 150

The body points are connected as shown. In all ailments it is important to connect G.V.20 to C.V.17. The Gov. Meridian controls all ordinary Yang Meridians +ve and the conception or Ren Meridian controls all ordinary Yin Meridians —ve. Therefore it is possible to obtain a balance.

The ear NT points are connected as shown, it is important that the two electrodes from the same terminal are not connected to the same ear.

Electro-acupuncture with WQ100 is always used for treatment of nervous tension.
Frequency: f_1 20 f_2 60.
Duration of treatment at least 60 mins each session treat weekly for 10-15 weeks.

Duration of treatment: At least 60 minutes each session. Treat weekly for 10-15 weeks.

For Schizophrenia: 5 needles must be used in the scalp G.V.20 — 1" Lateral and 1" Anterior and post to G.V.20 in addition to other points shown. Frequency: f_1 40 f_2 100 Hertz.

Endocrinology

1. Hormones controlling Breast Development and Function

2. Anatomy of the Breast

3. Lactation

4. Cosmetic - Acupuncture for Breast Development

5. Bone Pain - Malignant Hypercalcaemia

ENDOCRINOLOGY

ENDOCRINOLOGY
1. Lactation. 2. Cosmetic Acupuncture for Breast Development.
3. Bone Pain — Malignant Hypercalcaemia

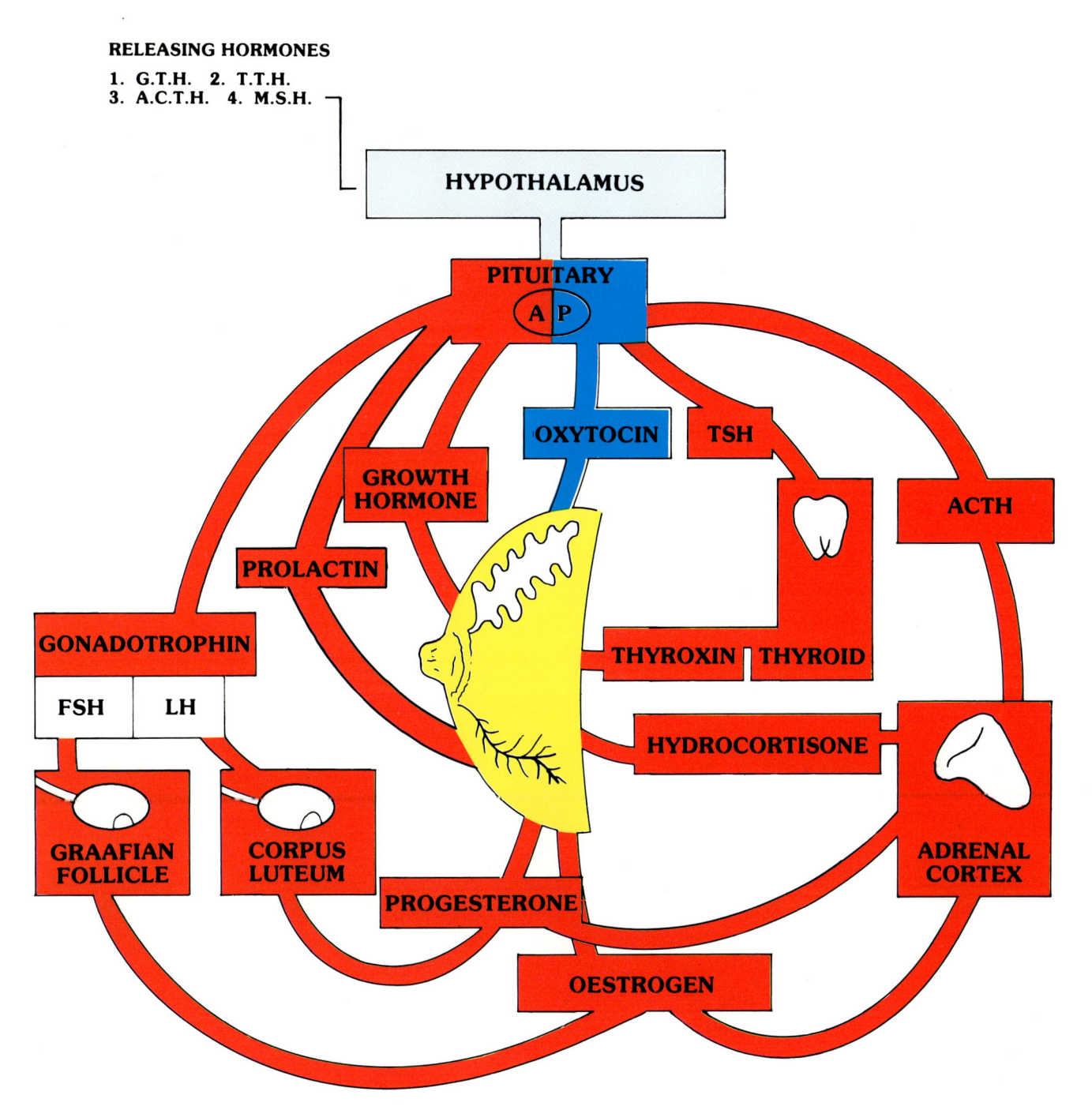

RELEASING HORMONES
1. G.T.H.   2. T.T.H.
3. A.C.T.H. 4. M.S.H.

Fig. 151

The above Diagram shows the Hormones acting on the Breast

ENDOCRINOLOGY

Anatomy of the Breast

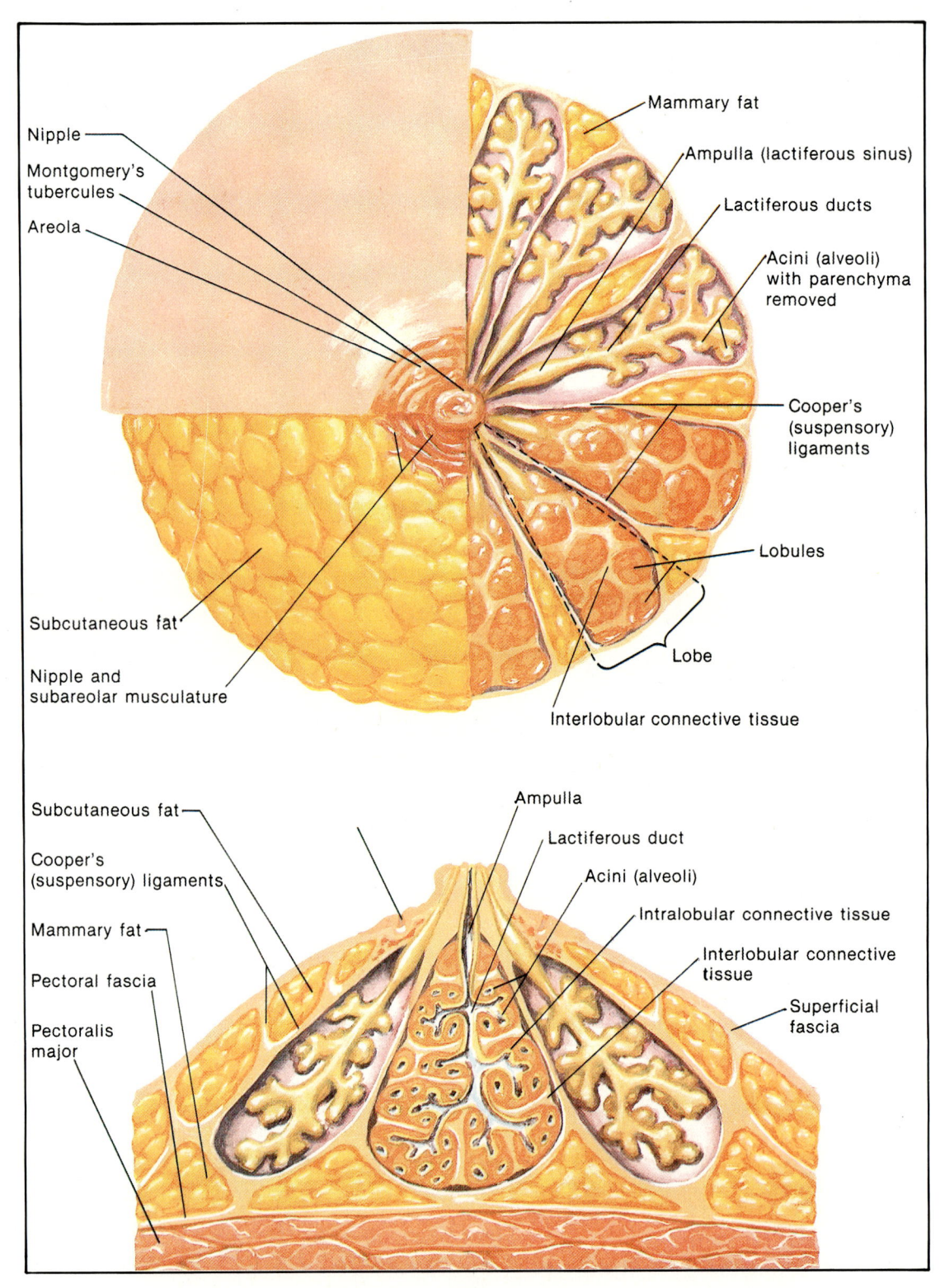

Fig. 152

with courtesy and kind permission of Ciba Geigy, Basle, Switzerland

ENDOCRINOLOGY

Vascular and Lymphatic Supply of the Breast

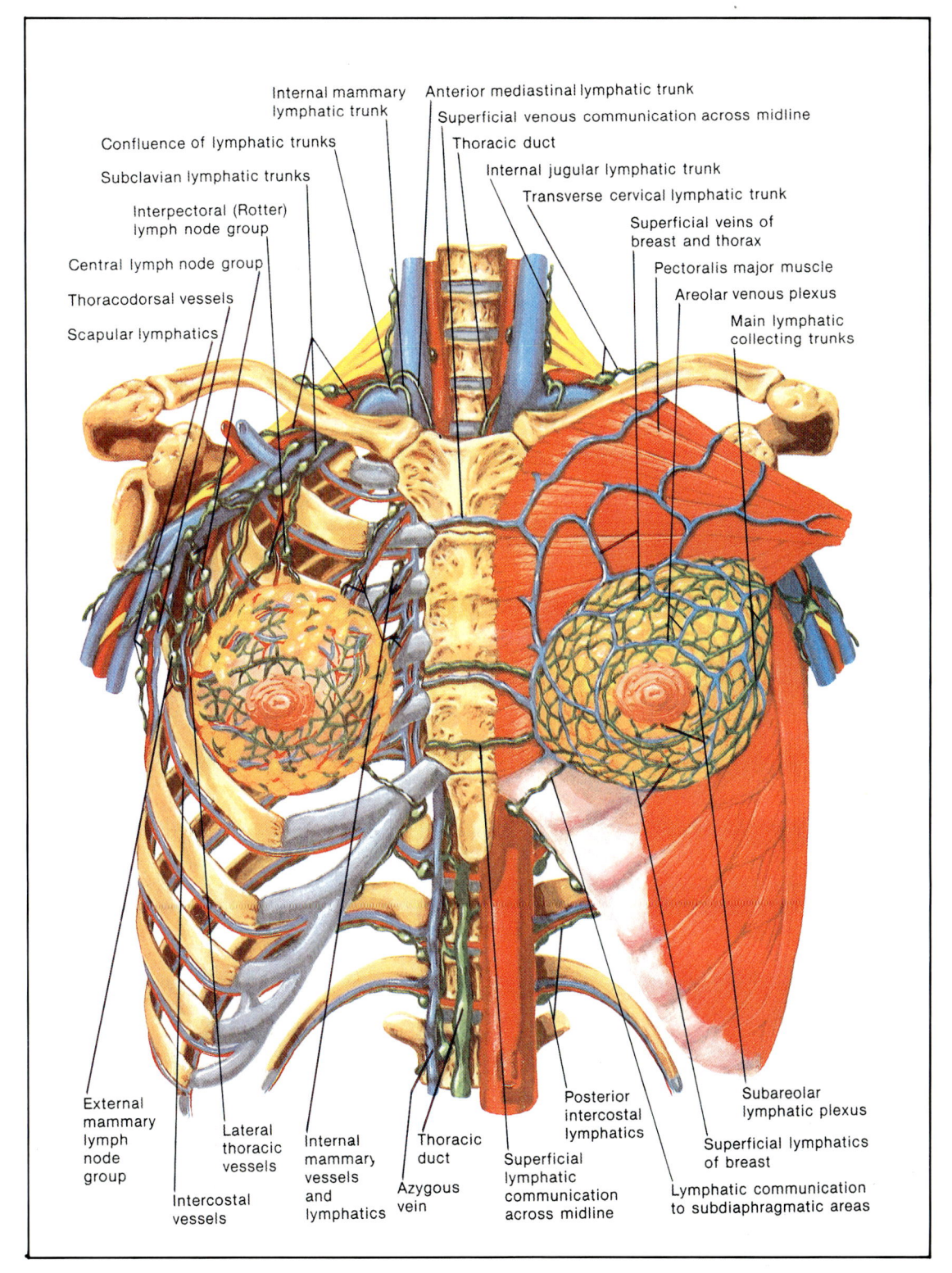

Fig. 153

with courtesy and kind permission of Ciba Geigy, Basle, Switzerland

ENDOCRINOLOGY

Fig. 154

- 4 Local Pts. around breast
- CV17
- CV15
- Co11
- CV10
- CV6
- TH5
- Co4
- St36
- Sp6
- Li3

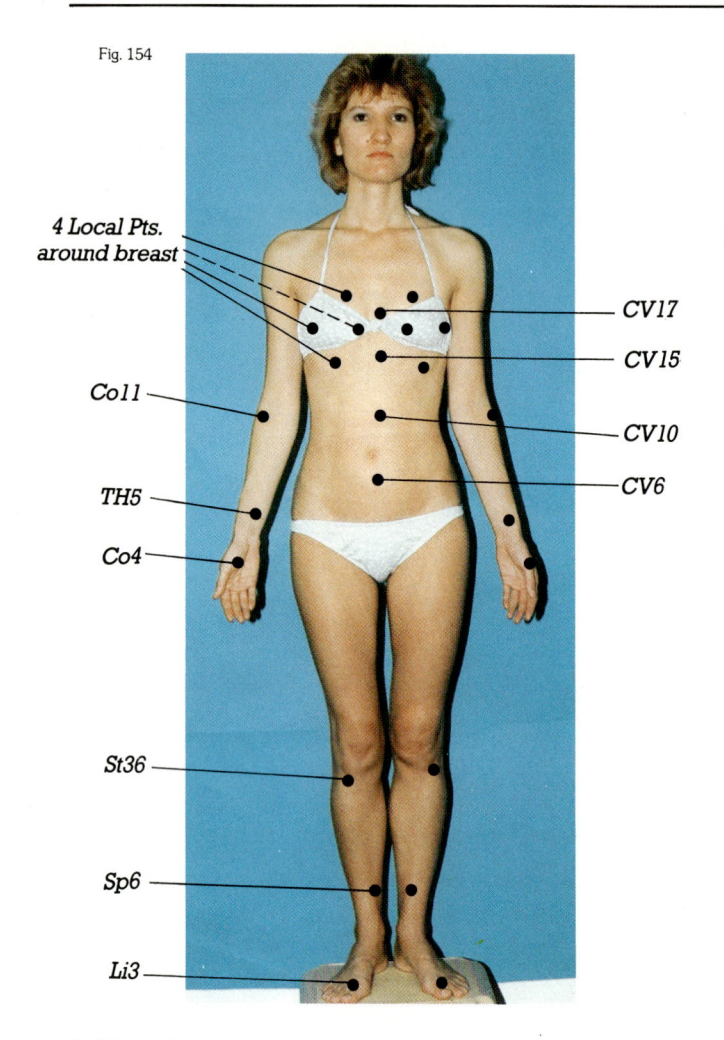

FOR COSMETIC ACUPUNCTURE

Body Pts. and ear Pts. are used as shown.

These are hormone points in ear and other relaxing points such as Anti-Aggression. Shenmen and also 4 local points in the breast.

Use 1″ needles for body and ½″ cosmetic 36 G for the ear. Connect bilaterally in both ears and also to body points.

ALWAYS USE ELECTRO-ACUPUNCTURE f_1 6 f_2 30 WQ100

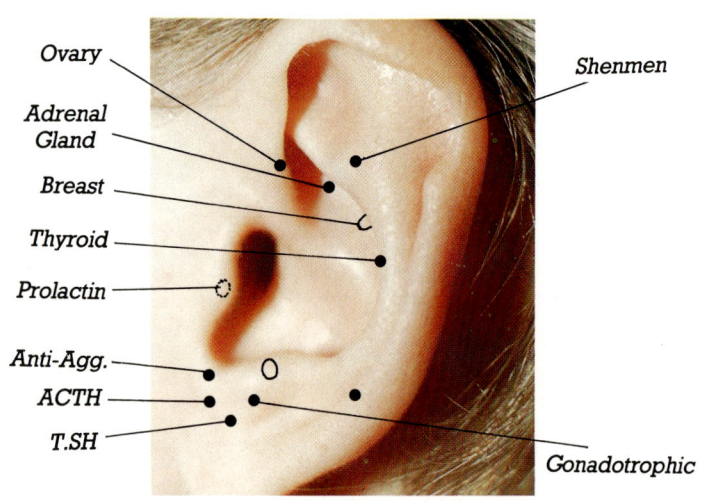

- Ovary
- Adrenal Gland
- Breast
- Thyroid
- Prolactin
- Anti-Agg.
- ACTH
- T.SH
- Shenmen
- Gonadotrophic

Fig. 155

MEERAN'S 12 NEEDLE TECHNIQUE FOR COSMETIC ACUPUNCTURE (BREAST DEVELOPMENT)

Stimulate points for 45-60 minutes twice weekly for 12 weeks.

BONE PAIN — MALIGNANT HYPERCALCAEMIA

Fig. 156

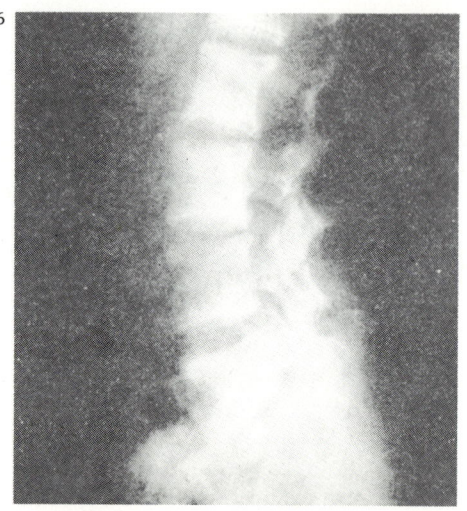

Metastatic Disease in Spine.

Fig. 157

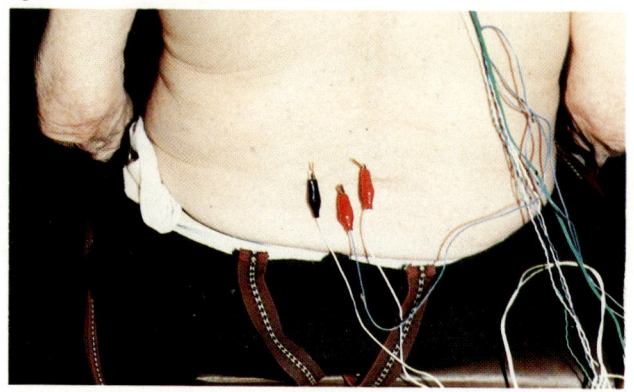

The normal blood Ca^{++} is 2.2-2.6 m mols/L. If above 3 m. mols/L.Pt. must be treated. Excess blood Ca^{++} can be due to Hyperparathyrodism, Vit D excess, sarcoidosis, Malignant conditions — Multiple Myeloma, secondaries from Ca Bronchus, Breast, Kidney, Thyroid, Prostate.

Symptoms: Bone Pain, Polydipsia, Polyuria, Mental Confusion, Weakness, Lethargy.

Always discuss case with ONCOLOGIST and RADIOTHERAPIST.

Aims of treatment: is (1) to make patient to have I.V. fluids to increase the Ca^{++} excretion in urine – distal tubule of Kidney. Hypercalcaemia is due to osteoclastic and osteoblastic activity by peptides produced by tumour or by inhibiting excretion of Ca^{++} by distal tubule. Calcitonin produced by calcitonin cells acts on distal tubule preventing reabsorption of Ca^{++}. Urinary Ca^{++} increases and blood Ca^{++} falls.

When this regime is followed patient's general condition improves due to reduction of serum calcium and also obtains pain relief.

1. BODY PTS IN SPINE

2. EAR PTS.

1. Calcitonin pt in Anti-Helix C_{6-7}
2. Shenmen.
3. ACTH and Anti-Aggression point.
4. Anti-Water Retention pt in Tragus
5. L. Sacral region for bone pain

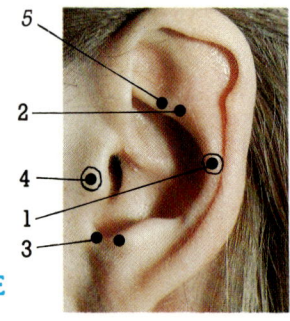

Fig. 158

Subfertility

1. General Facts on Subfertility
2. Diagram showing fertilisation of Ovum
3. Ear Points — Same points in both male and female
4. Body Points
5. Investigation of Subfertility

SUBFERTILITY

Subfertility is generally regarded as failure to conceive after some two years of unrestricted intercourse. It affects one couple in every ten. In two-thirds of cases one partner is responsible; in the remaining third the cause lies with both partners. It is a popular misconception that the problem is usually the woman's.

The normal course of events leading to pregnancy starts every month when one or other of the woman's ovaries sheds a ripe egg, usually about two weeks before her period is due. As shown in diagram, once released it enters a tube that connects the ovary to the womb, known as the fallopian tube. At the start of its journey along this tube the egg is ready for fertilisation. Should intercourse occur at this stage the sperm, initially deposited at the mouth of the womb, will swim up into the fallopian tubes by chemical attraction. When they reach the egg, fertilisation can occur if one sperm successfully penetrates it. If this happens the egg, formerly just one cell, divides repeatedly to form a ball of cells called the morula. Meanwhile the ball is still travelling down the tube towards the womb. Once there, the ball of cells becomes a hollow sphere with a mound of cells on one part of the inner surface. In successful conception this sphere must embed itself into the wall of the womb, where it receives food and oxygen from what becomes the placenta.

There are many things that can prevent this normal conception occurring; before subfertility can be treated the cause must be identified. The first stage towards this is to investigate both partners. The doctor needs to know both their own and their family's medical history. He will also look for signs and symptoms of subfertility.

In the case of the woman, age may be a factor, for female fertility naturally declines after the age of twenty-five. Other indications are irregular ovulation, physical abnormalities in the genital tract, hormone imbalance, blockage in the fallopian tubes and pelvic infections, including tuberculosis. Personality problems affecting libido can also be important.

When he examines the man, the physician is once again on the lookout for physical abnormalities in the reproductive organs. He will also check the quality and quantity of sperm in the seminal fluid. There may be an unusually high proportion of malformed sperm, or the total number present may be considerably lower than the normal 300 to 400 million per ejaculation. Hormonal imbalance and problems of impotency and premature ejaculation are also important factors.

In approximately ten per cent of subfertile couples the man's sperm is incompatible with the mucus at the neck of the woman's womb (the cervix), so preventing the sperm from reaching the fallopian tubes. This shared problem may be due to sperm defects, thick or insufficient cervical mucus, or sperm antibodies. In the latter case, the man, the woman or both may have antibodies against sperms which prevent them from penetrating the cervical mucus. If this is happening a microscopic examination of the mixture of sperm and mucus shows the sperms characteristically immobilised and clumped into groups. Individual sperm may show a shaking movement but are usually unable to move forwards.

After the initial investigation of both partners, the next stage is to set up an accurate record of the woman's menstrual cycle, for whoever is responsible for the lack of conception, the doctor needs to know the cycle length and the time of ovulation so that, problems aside, he knows the cycle length and the time conceiving. The accepted way to do this is to tell the woman to record her body temperature every morning on a temperature chart and in addition to keep a note of the days she has intercourse. By analysing the changes in temperature the doctor can ascertain her fertile phase, the optimum time for conception. A small drop in temperature followed by a clear rise marks the release of an egg from the ovary. If conception does not occur the temperature remains high until her period occurs, after which it falls.

Some cases of subfertility are not suitable for acupuncture therapy; the doctor can determine this in his initial diagnosis. Luckily most subfertile couples can be treated very successfully using acupuncture in a combined treatment with fertility drugs. The acupuncture side of the treatment lasts from six to twelve week, depending on severity, with either one or two sessions per week.

Where the woman appears to be the cause she is prescribed fertility drugs like clomid or bromocriptine. Her acupuncture therapy involves the use of body points and ear points. The main body points are Spleen Six, above the ankle joint, and two points in the abdominal wall, one above and one below the naval. Both points lie along the Conception Vessel meridian. Of the three major ear points used, one specifically affects the hormone balance.

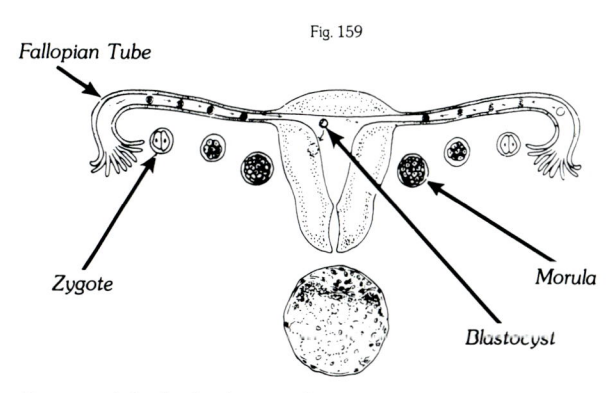

Fig. 159

Passage of the fertilised egg to the womb.

EAR POINTS

Fig. 160

SUBFERTILITY

POINTS FOR SUBFERTILITY IS THE SAME FOR BOTH SEXES.

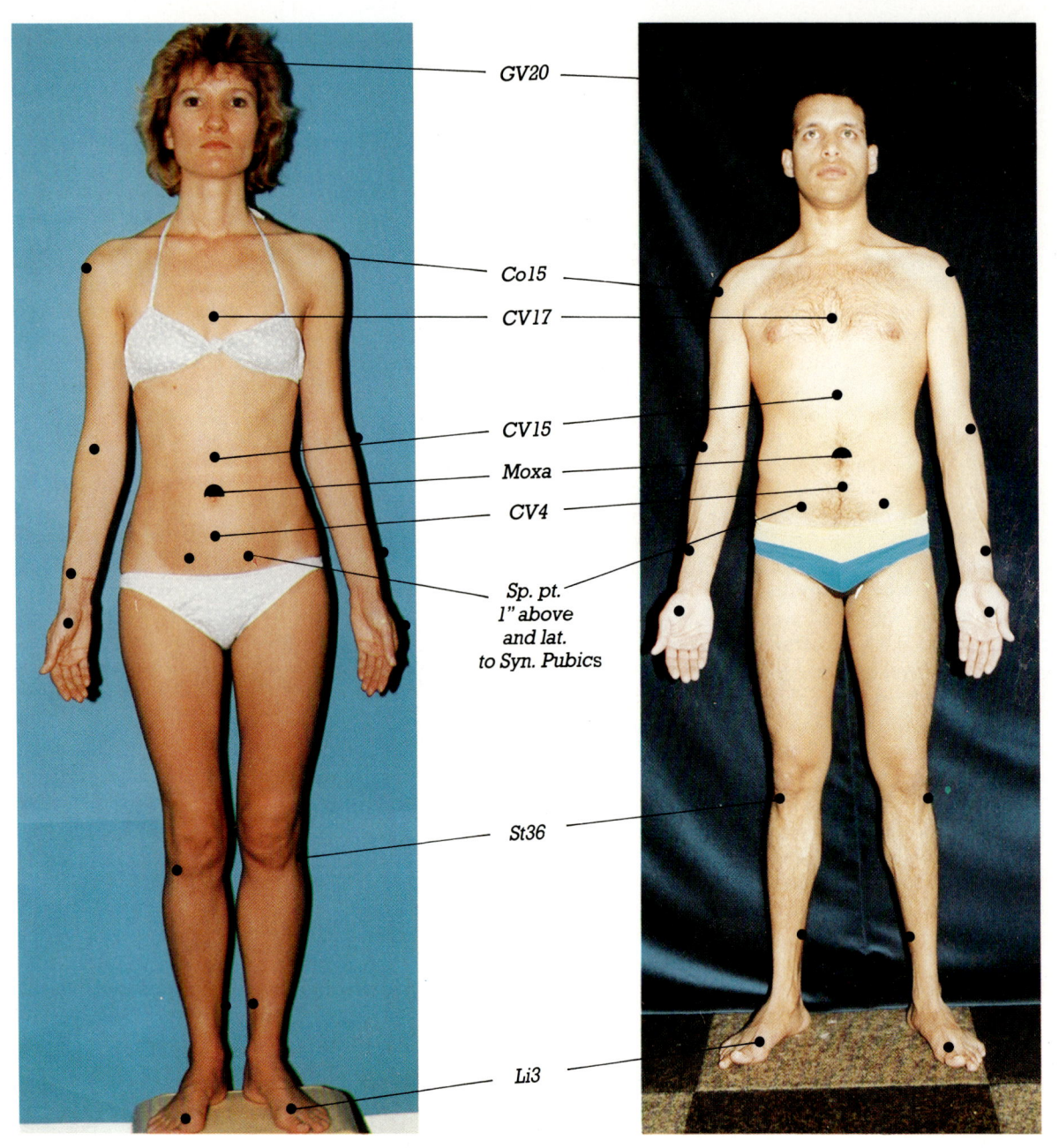

Labels on Fig. 161 and Fig. 162: GV20, Co15, CV17, CV15, Moxa, CV4, Sp. pt. 1" above and lat. to Syn. Pubics, St36, Li3

Fig. 161

Fig. 162

1. Body and Ear Points are shown.
2. **INVESTIGATE BOTH PARTNERS ALWAYS.**
   a. Patency of tubes and hormone assay etc in female.
   b. Sperm count morphology, mobility of sperm essential.
   c. Post Coital test.

Stimulate all points bilaterally with electro-acupuncture. Treat one or both partners depending on investigations. Treat once a week for 12 weeks. Each session 45 minutes minimum.

If the man needs treatment, he undergoes a very similar course of therapy. Instead of clomiphene or bromocriptine, the man with a low sperm count is given male hormones called androgens in combination with fairly large doses of Vitamin E, or Anti-Oestrogenic preperations like tamoxifen.

The acupuncture side of his treatment involves the same body points: Spleen Six, above the ankle, and the two Conception Vessel points, above and below the navel. In the ear, points corresponding to the testes and the prostrate gland are needled and stimulated in addition to the Shenmen point and an extra point just below the ear, known as the ACTH point. This point stimulates the release of Adrenocortico Trophic Hormone.

The man's sperm count should increase with this treatment. When this happens conception is still more likely if his seminal fluid is used to artificially inseminate the woman. Ideally this is done on day 14 of a 28-day menstrual cycle. If the woman's cycle is shorter or longer than this, the time of insemination is adjusted accordingly.

Subfertility is a long-term condition and acupuncture is ideal for its treatment because the effects of needle stimulation are continuous between sessions. The success rates of acupuncture therapy for subfertility reflect this, for they are far higher than when drugs alone are used.

Psycho-Sexual Problems

1. **Impotence**
2. **Frigidity**
3. **Dyspareunia**

PSYCHO-SEXUAL PROBLEMS

IMPOTENCE — FRIGIDITY — DYSPAREUNIA

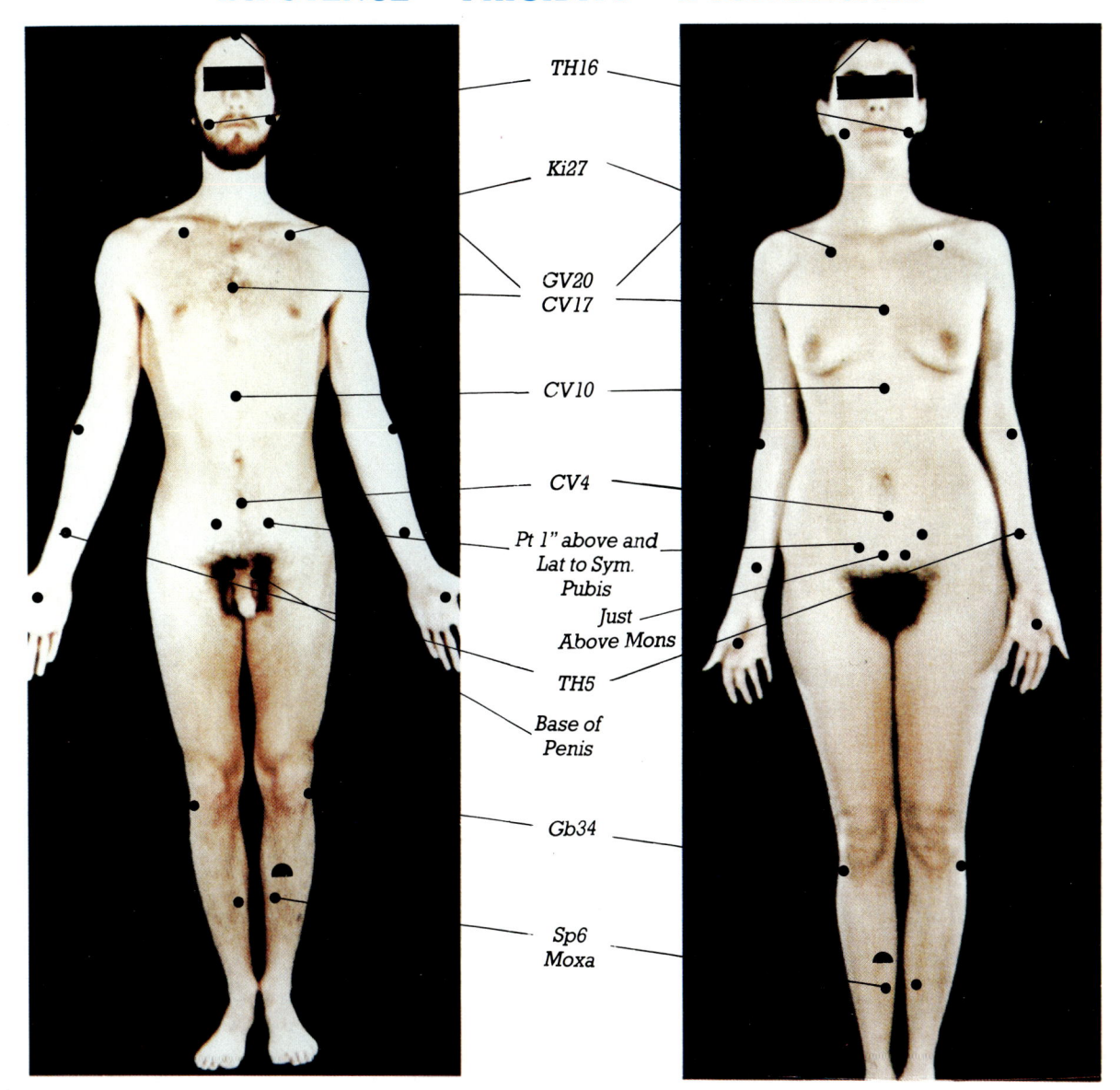

Fig. 163

Fig. 164

Many patients with impotence or frigidity have no definable organic cause.

1. Careful history, physical disease, stress and **psychological factors.**
   Drugs — Methyl Dopa, Cimetidine, Spironolactone, CNS depressants, Combined Oral Contraceptives, Clonidine, Antihistamines etc, Beta Blockers, Alcohol.

2. Medical conditions such as Diabetes Mellitus, Hyperthyroidism, Drugs.
   Endocrine causes are those of Hypogonadism - must be excluded.
   By 1. Normal Testosterone.
       2. Gonadotrophins.
       3. Prolactin levels.

Autonomic Neuropathy — most commonly from Diabetes Mellitus — is the commonest identifiable cause.

Acupuncture will help in the majority of cases of impotence and frigidity if psycho-sexual. But treatment must be consistent and regularly done.

For both conditions similar points are used —
— Body Points
— Ear Points
— Special Points.

Always use Electro-Acupuncture with WQ100 or IC-1107 Electro-Acupunctoscope.

BODY POINTS ARE SHOWN

Connect electrodes as indicated in figure 163, 164.

Three Heater Point TH_{16} TH_5
Spleen 6

A point on either side of the base of the penis and another point 1" above and lateral to this point is important.

Moxa or Maruku-Ban is used at Spleen 6 and umbilicus daily. Patient must be given the proper instruction.

Maruku-Ban — 20-30 minutes. Caution: Explain to patient regarding thermal burns if kept long.

EAR POINTS: Important points are Bosch Pt. Penis or clitoris point GTH, prefrontal cortex — as it controls emotions. Shenmen.

Electro-acupuncture: 45 minutes twice a week for 6-8 weeks.

PSYCHO-SEXUAL PROBLEMS

DYSPAREUNIA: Exclude organic causes, use the Special Point in the Mesenchaeilon below Ext. Auditory Meatus below point for muscle tone (Fig. 85). Also use NT pt. of Body and Ear.

Ear points for Impotence and Frigidity

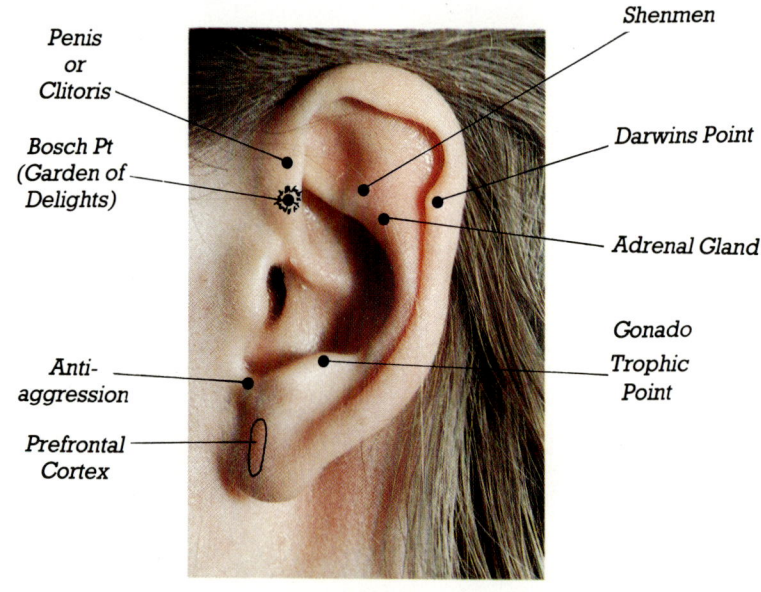

Penis or Clitoris
Bosch Pt (Garden of Delights)
Anti-aggression
Prefrontal Cortex
Shenmen
Darwins Point
Adrenal Gland
Gonado Trophic Point

Fig. 165

Body points for Impotence

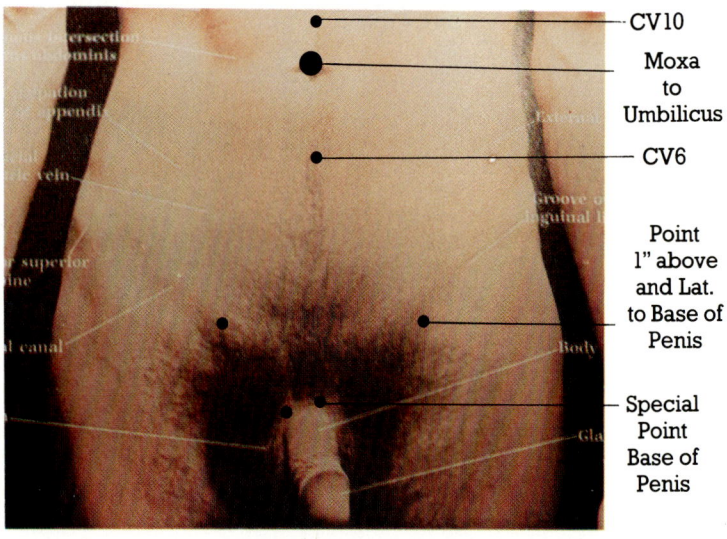

CV10 — Moxa to Umbilicus
CV6
Point 1" above and Lat. to Base of Penis
Special Point Base of Penis

Fig. 166

Dyspareunia - is pain during sexual intercourse. Exclude organic causes, e.g. Pelvic inflamation, Fibroids, retroverted Uterus etc.
In many cases it is functional.

Body Points used: — Nervous Tension Points
G.V. 20 C.V. 17 Co_4 Co_{11} Co_{15} TH_{16} Li_3 Sp_6 St_{36}

Connect points bilaterally, Body and Ear points.
Frequency 20 Hertz.
Treatment — 30 mins - weekly for 4 weeks.

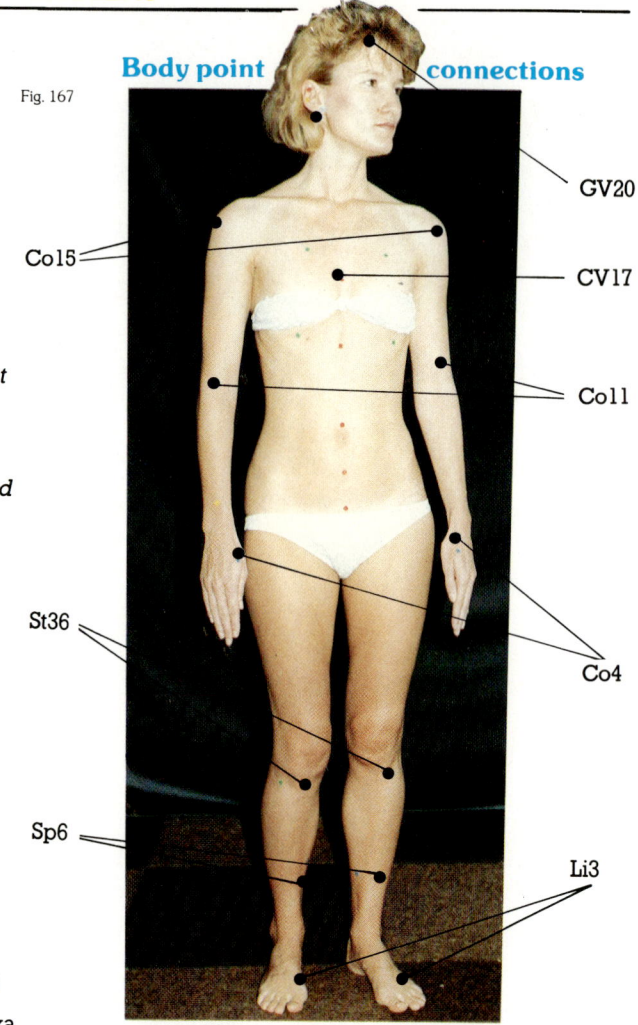

Body point connections

Fig. 167

GV20, Co15, CV17, Co11, St36, Co4, Sp6, Li3

Body points - Nervous Tension points

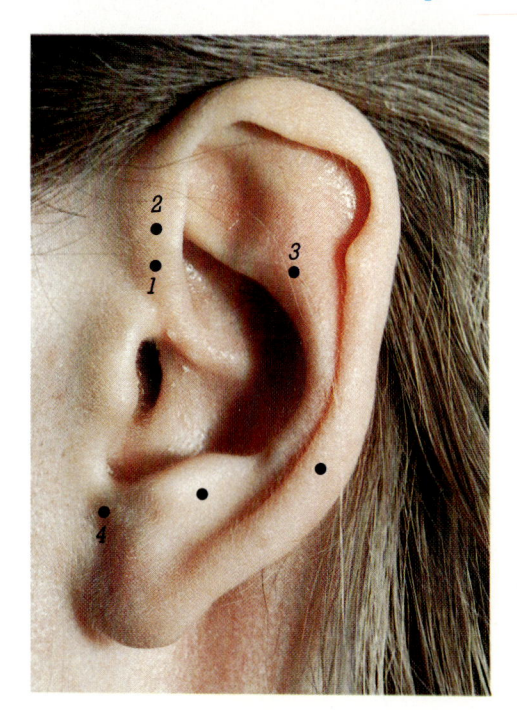

Fig. 168

Ear Points for Dyspareunia

1. Bosch point 2. Clitoris 3. Shenmen
4. Anti-Aggression 5. Anti-Tragus
6. Point of Jerome

108

Nose Acupuncture

Hand Acupuncture

Foot Acupuncture

NOSE ACUPUNCTURE

Acupuncture treatment until recently has been concentrated on:—
- BODY ACUPUNCTURE
- MERIDIAN THEORY
- AURICULAR ACUPUNCTURE
- LASER ACUPUNCTURE
- SCALP or HEAD ACUPUNCTURE

In this section of the Atlas the following will be dealt with:—
1. Nose Acupuncture
2. Hand Acupuncture
3. Foot Acupuncture

All the above are developed from.
1. The Meridian Theory.
2. Many diseases can be treated with the use of one single Acupuncture point.

For example in hand acupuncture - the chest point which shown can be used for treating chest pain, Intercostal Neuralgia, but also for Epilepsy and Vomiting.

However even though they work, much research is still necessary to explain how these points work on Anatomy, Neuro-Physiology and Medical Grounds.

3. Location of points must be very accurate.

4. If necessary, body, ear acupuncture points and moxibustion can be used in combination ex. for Hyperhidrosis - point in palm of hand in centre of palm and Sympathetic point in ear, heart 7 and Pericadium 6 in body acupuncture.

NOSE ACUPUNCTURE

According to the theory of Chinese medicine, the nose is situated in the middle of the face and therefore becomes the meeting point for Blood and Chi (Energy of Life) of the whole body. It is also the starting point for all Cardio-Pulmonary function.

Nose acupuncture points are formed in a line system. There are three lines found on the nose - with the second and third lines formed in corresponding pairs.

Points on the Nose and their location - 38 points on Nose

Fig. 169

- Head and Neck
- Throat
- Lung
- Heart
- Liver
- Spleen
- Kidney
- External Genital Organ

Line 1. — From this one third of forehead to the tip of the Philtrum forming the midline of the nose.

Solid organs in midline of the nose, the 8 points are shown in the figure.

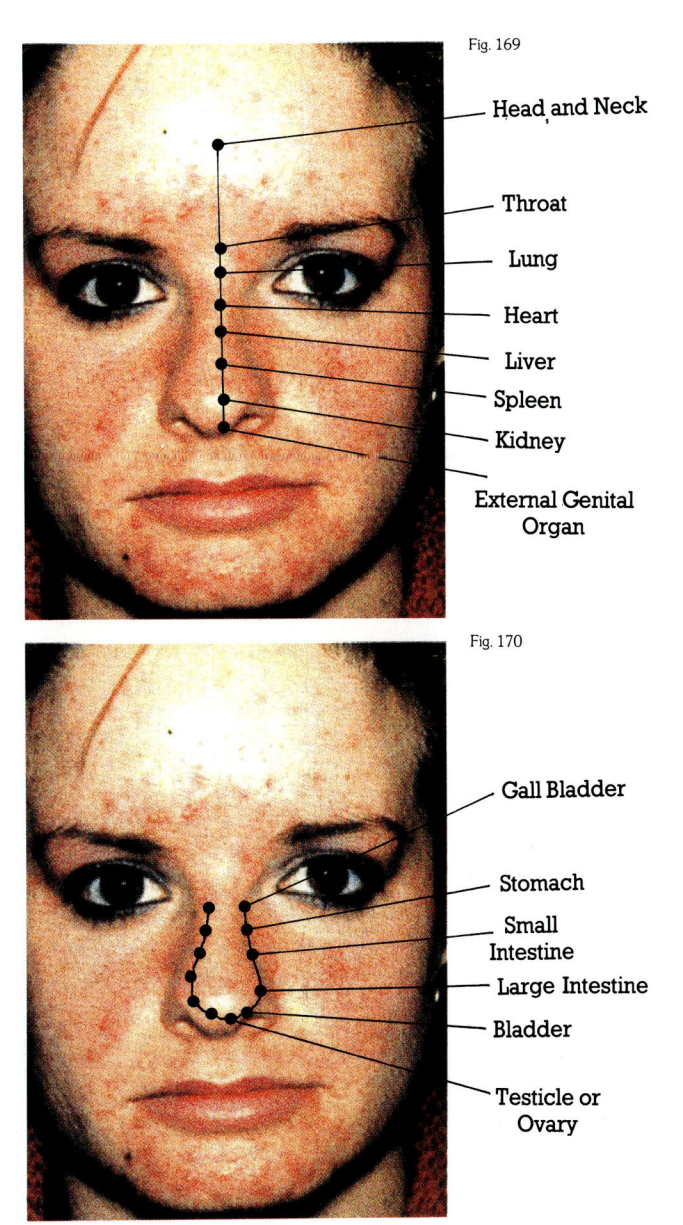

Line 2. — Hollow organs 10 points on second line. Line 2 is close to the midline following the contour of the nose commencing beside the liver point and terminating at the lower border of the Ala Nasi.

Fig. 170

- Gall Bladder
- Stomach
- Small Intestine
- Large Intestine
- Bladder
- Testicle or Ovary

Line 3. — 18 points at the third line. From the medial end of the eyebrows to the Ala Nasi - lateral sides of the second chest extremities situated at both lateral sides of line 2. Points are ear, chest, breast, nape, loin, upper limb, thigh, knee, foot and toe.

HAND & FOOT ACUPUNCTURE

The 18 points at the third lines are shown

INDICATION and NEEDLING

As stated earlier, nose acupuncture needling can be combined with body or ear acupuncture.

Points are chosen according to their nature and to correspond to which organ or system is deseased.

It is better to combine nose points and meridian points to obtain the best results.

Needling

Select the appropriate point and the following needle technique is used:—

1. If the point selected falls on the first or second line, oblique or horizontal needle technique is used.
2. If on the third line, oblique or vertical insertion can be used.
3. Duration of Treatment:— 20 mins - use 2 or 3 sessions a week till symptoms improve.

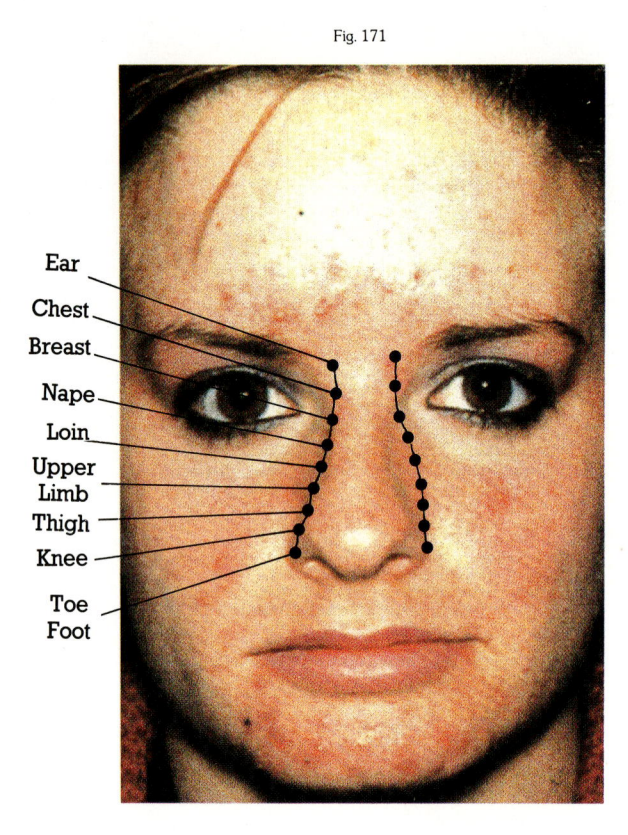

Fig. 171

Hand and Foot Acupuncture

Only the important points are shown on the Dorsum of hand and foot - including the nail points.

HAND AND FOOT ACUPUNCTURE

Hand and foot acupuncture is the insertion of needles in certain points in the hand or foot so that various diseases can be cured, usually good for acute pain.

The meridian points in the hand or foot are very useful and must be known very well.

Hand and foot acupuncture is not used very much and only the important points will be shown on the dorsum of the hand and foot.

HAND ACUPUNCTURE

1. Hand relaxed and slightly flexed.
2. ½ to 1 inch needle used.
3. Needle inserted 15% - depth 0.41 inches.

FOOT ACUPUNCTURE

1. Choose relavent point required for treatment.
2. Points chosen in pairs.
3. Needle inserted for depth ½ inch with moderate stimulation. Duration 3 to 5 minutes.

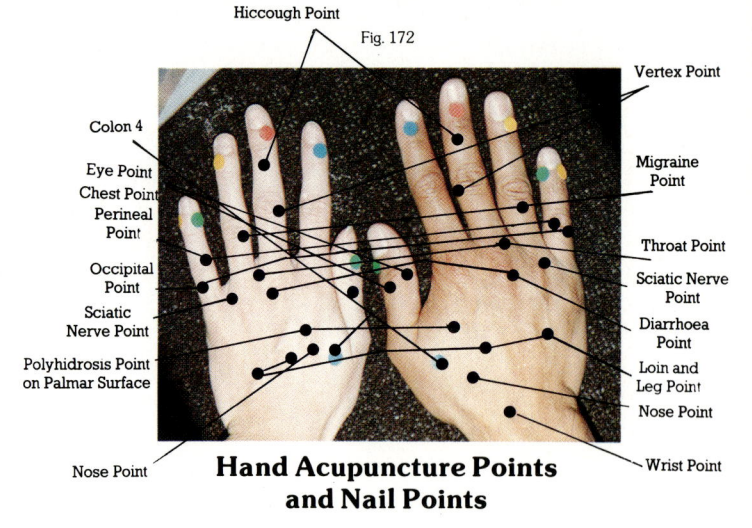

Hand Acupuncture Points and Nail Points

Fig. 172

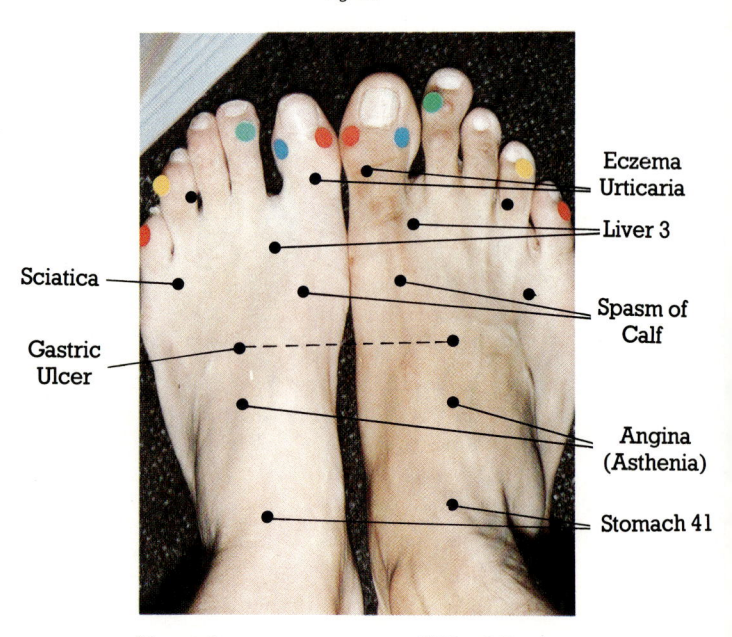

Foot Acupuncture and Nail Points

Fig. 173

Scalp or Head Acupuncture

1. **Division of Stimulation Areas**
2. **Localisation of Motor Area**
3. **Functional Localisation**
4. **Stimulation Areas in Skull Acupuncture**
5. **Selection of points and methods of Manipulation**

SCALP OR HEAD ACUPUNCTURE

Division of Stimulation Areas

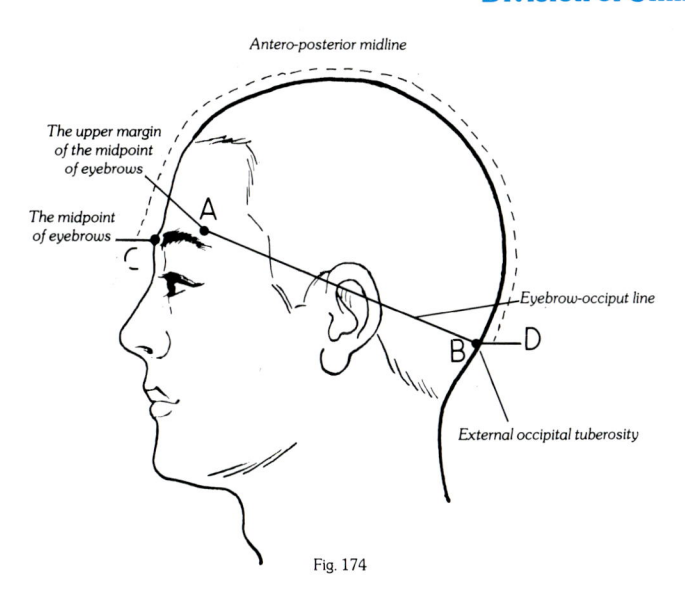

Fig. 174

Stimulation Area of Scalp-Needle Standard lines

Two standard lines Midline CD and Eyebrow Occiput AB are drawn to divide the stimulation areas.

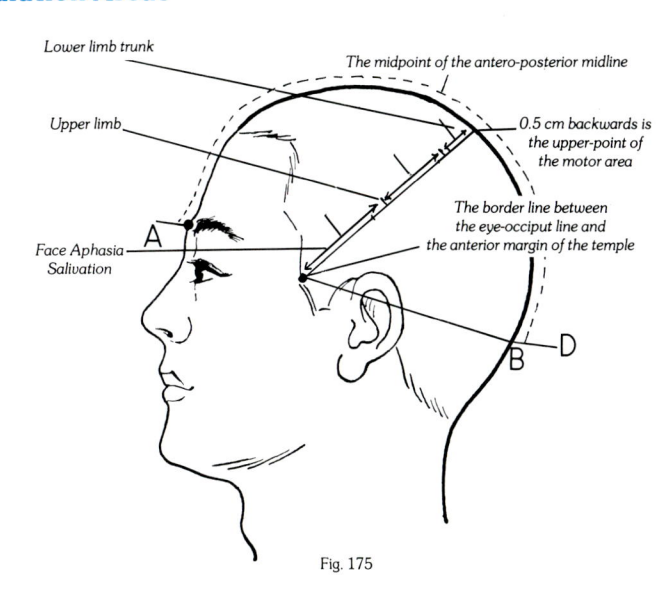

Fig. 175

Localization of Motor Area

Upper 1 fifth Lower Limb, Trunk
Middle 2 fifths Upper Limb
Lower 2 fifths face, Aphasia, Salivation, Aphonla.

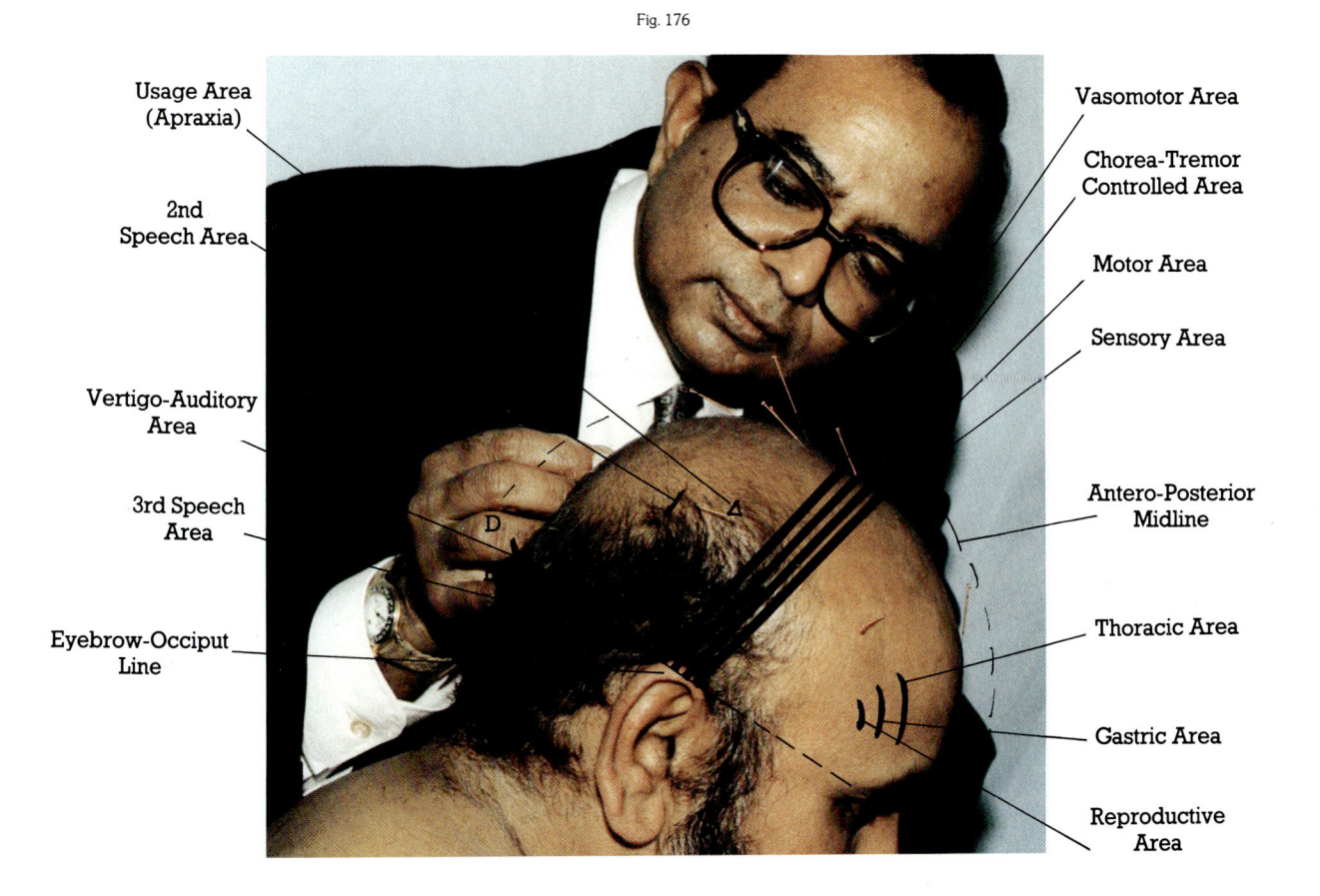

Fig. 176

Standard lines AB, CD shown
Stimulation areas shown on scalp:—
Sensory, Motor Chorea - Tremor area and vaso motor areas shown in middle of scalp.
Thoracic, Gastric and Reproductive areas shown lateral to midline.
Vertigo - Auditory area, usage area shown above pinna.
and demonstration of needle insertion in face sensory area

SCALP OR HEAD ACUPUNCTURE

SCALP NEEDLING THERAPY

Acupuncture on the scalp was worked out by a physician - Chiao Shun - F A and his colleagues in a north China County Hospital.

Used to treat paralysis caused by brain diseases.

The determination of the main part of stimulation areas in scalp needling depends upon the projection by the gyrus and sulcus on the cerebral hemisphere.

Functional localisation of the cerebral cortex must be fully understood in the use of scalp needling.

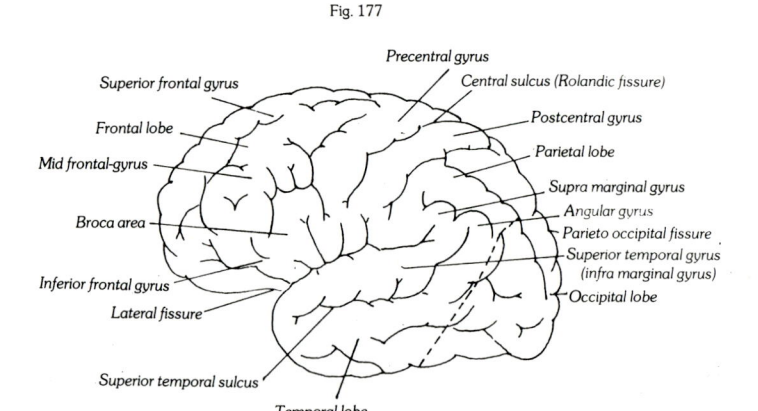

Fig. 177

Lateral Surface of the Left Cerebral Hemisphere

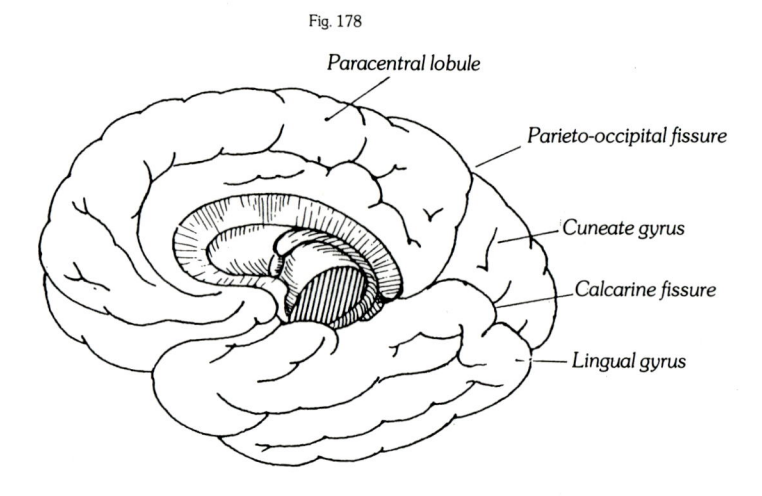

Fig. 178

Medial Surface of the Right Cerebral Hemisphere

Before Therapy:—

1. Full history and examination.
2. Nervous System, Motor sensory, reflexes, cranial nerves.
3. Gait.
4. Investigations must be done.

Selection of Points and Methods of Manipulation

1. Disease in unilateral limb, select stimulation area on the contra-lateral side.

2. Bilateral disease, use bilateral stimulation.

3. For Hypertension, vertigo limb numbness, urticaria and for disease where focus cannot be distinguished, use bilateral stimulation.

4. If there are complicated symptoms for example in paralysis of the lower limb - needling of the motor area may be combined with the foot motor sensory area.

MANIPULATION

1. Sterilize the region of the scalp which is to be needled.

2. Insert 2 - 3 inch needle gauge 32 into the stimulation area under the skin - by twisting and turning the needle. The needle must be absolutely fixed.

3. Twisting the needle in the frequency of 200 times per minute or electro-acupuncture with WQ 100 electronic acupunctoscope or IC-1107 Electro-Acupunctoscope.

4. Generally after 1 minute of stimulation, the corresponding limb or internal organ will get a feeling of heat, numbness, soreness etc.

5. Continue stimulation for 5 mins., then rest for 5 to 10 minutes.

6. Repeat stimulation 3-4 times. Then withdraw needles.

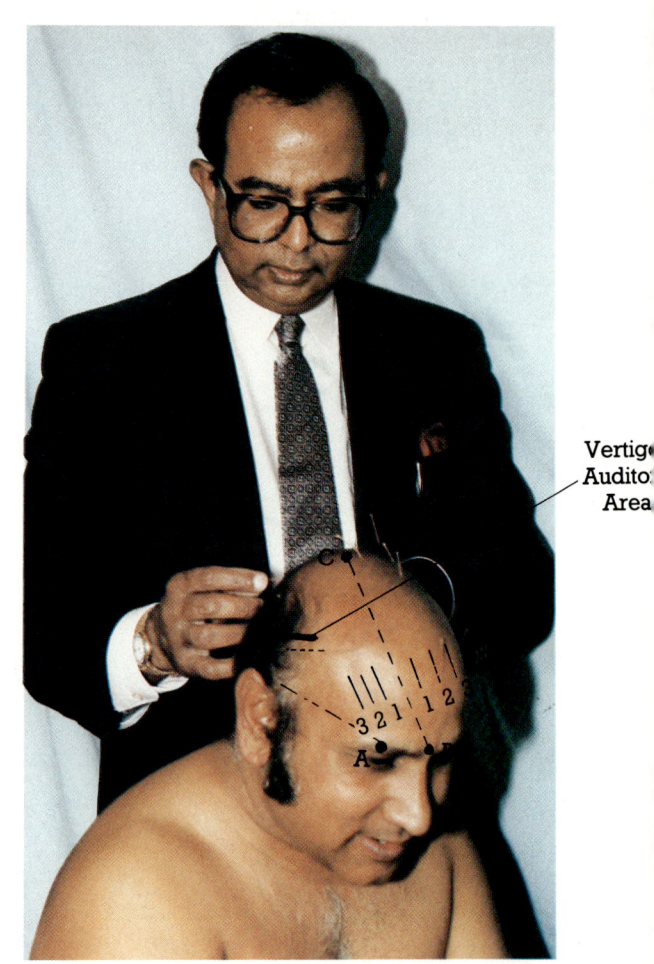

Fig. 179

1. Thoracic Area 2. Gastric Area 3. Reproductive Area
Demonstration of needle in balance area - accurate localisation of point is required.

SCALP OR HEAD ACUPUNCTURE

Stimulation Areas in Skull Acupuncture

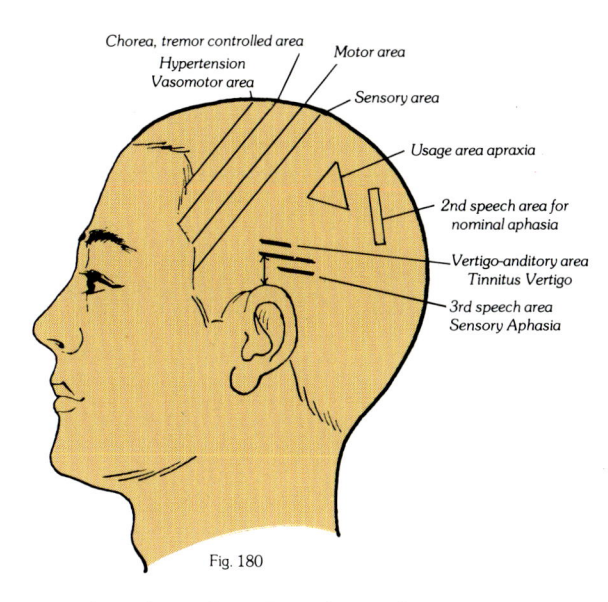

Fig. 180

Lateral Surface of the Stimulation Areas

MOTOR AREA 0.5 c.m. behind Mid. Point
Upper 1 fifth Lower Limb, Trunk area
Middle 2 fifths Upper Limb
Lower 2 fifths Face Area

SENSORY AREA 1.5 c.m. behind Motor Area
Upper 1 fifth Contralat, Lumbago, Pain Lower Limb
Numbness, Occipital Headache, Vertigo

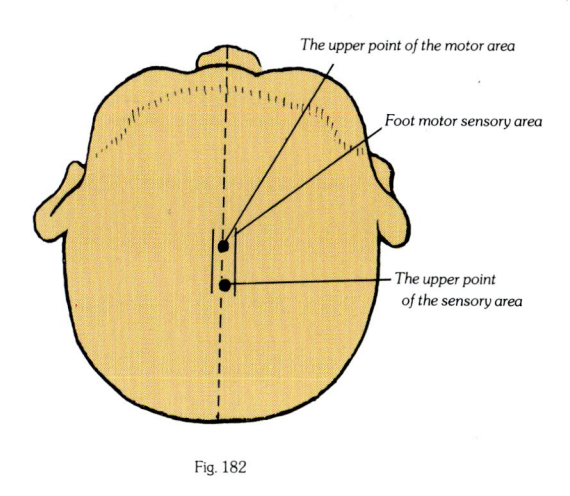

Fig. 182

Parietal Surface of the Stimulation Areas

Middle 2 fifths - Contra - Lateral Pain Numbness and Upper Limb
Lower 2 fifths - Contralateral, Trigeminal Neuralgia, Toothache, Tempero-Mandibular Arthritis.

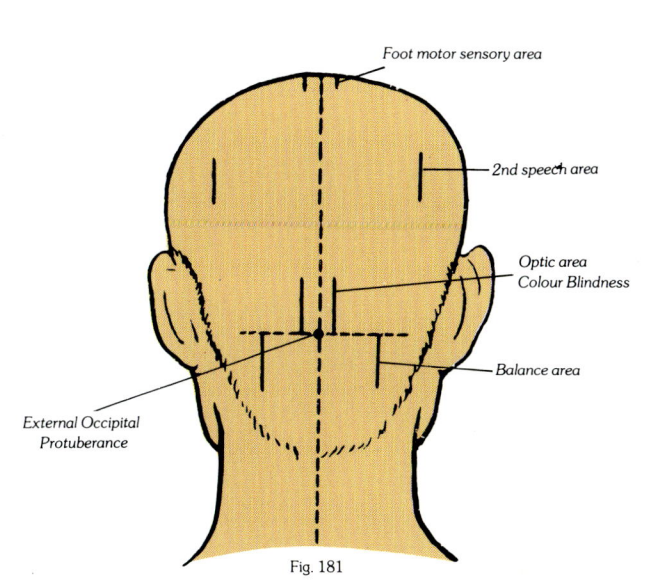

Fig. 181

Posterior Surface of the Stimulation Areas

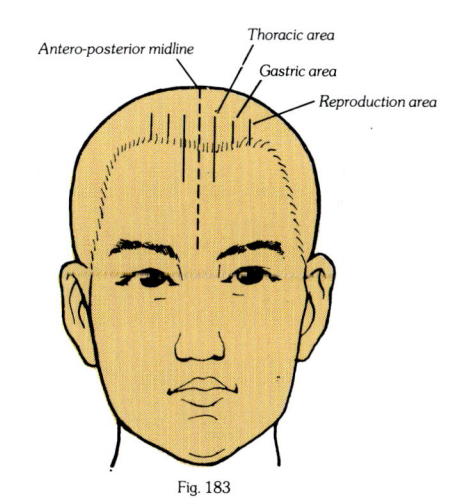

Fig. 183

Anterior Surface of the Stimulation areas

OPTIC AREA - Draw a line 1 c.m. from the Ext. Occ. Protuberance 4 cms. long. Used for Colour Blindness.

BALANCE AREA - Draw a line 4 cms. long - 3 cms. below Ext. Occ. Protuberance. Used for unstable balance caused by Cerebeller Disease.

REPRODUCTIVE AREA - Lateral to Gastric area 2 cm. line in line lat border of Eye Brow for Dysfunctional Uterine Bleeding, Dysmenorrhoea, Dyspareunia.

GASTRIC AREA - Hair line and in line of pupil draw a line 2 cms. parallel to A. P. Line used for Epigastric Discomfort.

THORACIC AREA - Between Gastric Area and A.P. line 4 cms. long - used for Asthma, Chest Ailments, Supra Ventricular Proxysmal Tachycardia.

Miscellaneous Facts and Treatments

1. Needles used for stimulating ear with electro-acupunpuncture before using semi-permanent needle.

2. Molybdenum needle inserted at zero point of Nogier

3. Semi-permanent needle ring and stem type being inserted into ear (auricle)

4. Herpes zoster in a 7 year old girl - very rare at this age.

5. Inserting a needle at GV20 - mid-point of the scalp (Bahuj - GV20)

6. Treatment of Raynaud's disease - needles at S.I.2, Ht. 7 - electro-stimulation

7. Marukyu Ban thermal plasters being used for backache with needles

8. Treatment of Arthritis of the knee. IC 1103 was used for electro-stimulation

9. Treatment of Post-Hepatic Neuralgia Herpes Zoster about 2 years ago. Patient still having pain L 6th and 7th thoracic nerves involved - 3 sessions with electro-acupuncture successfully treated.

MISCELLANEOUS FACTS AND TREATMENTS

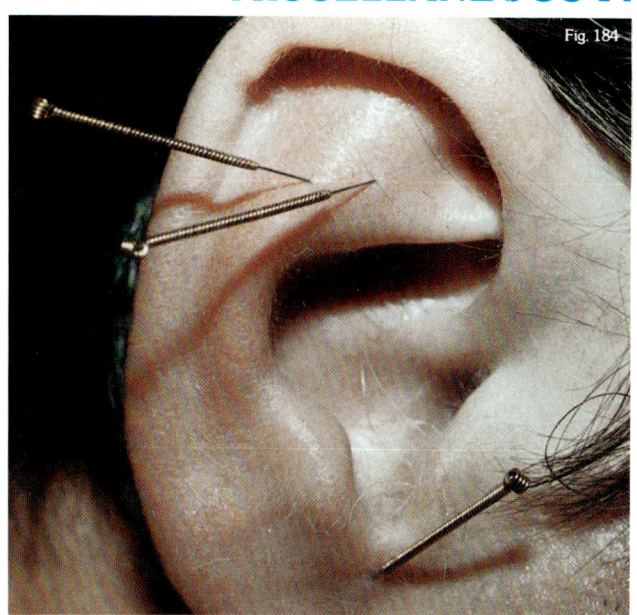

Fig. 184

Needles used for stimulating ear with electro-acupuncture. Before using semi-permanent needles.

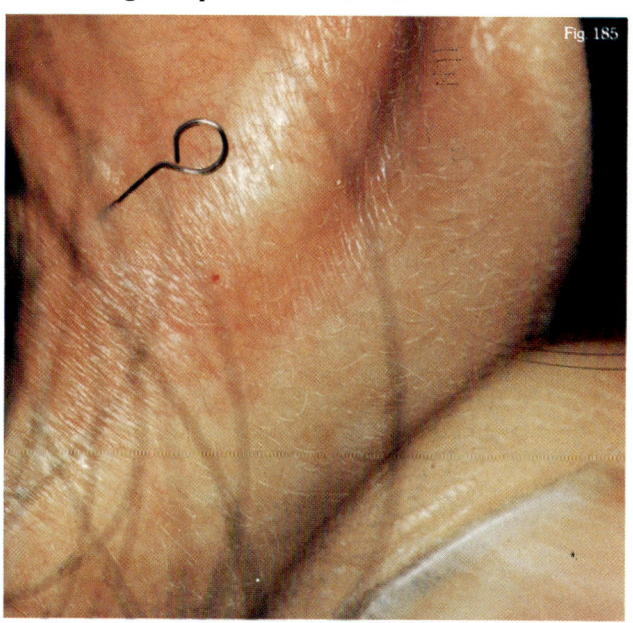

Fig. 185

Semi permanent needle, ring and stem type being inserted into ear (Auricle).

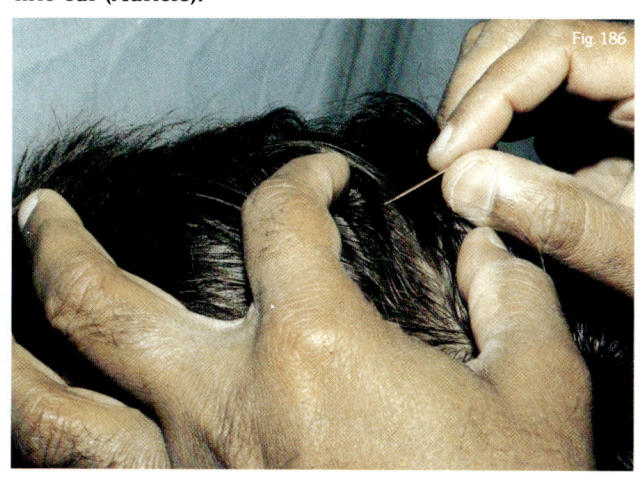

Fig. 186

Inserting a needle at G.V.20 mid point of the scalp (Bahui — G.V.20).

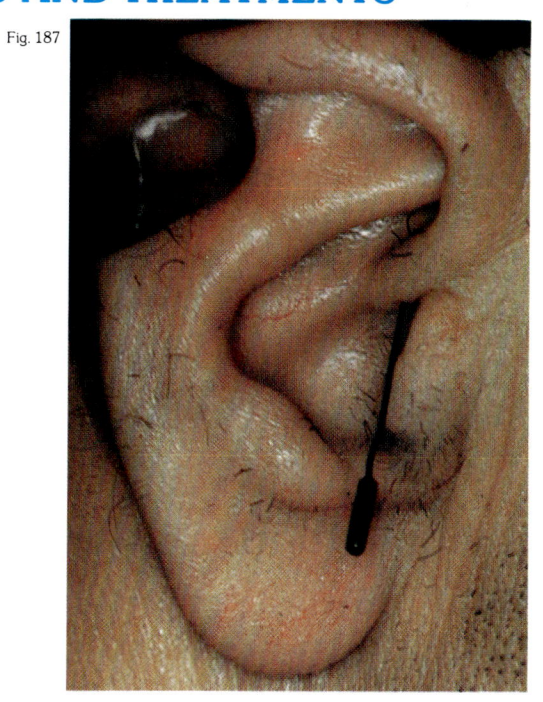

Fig. 187

Molybdenum needle inserted at Zero Point of Nogier.

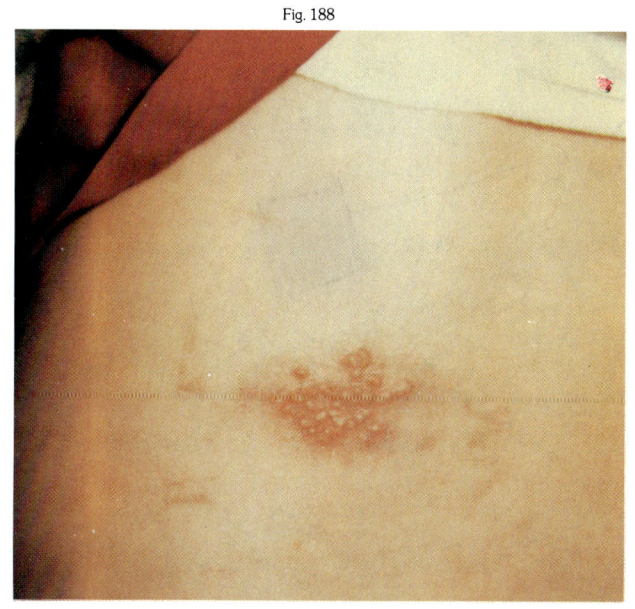

Fig. 188

Herpes zoster in a 7-year-old girl. Very rare at this age.

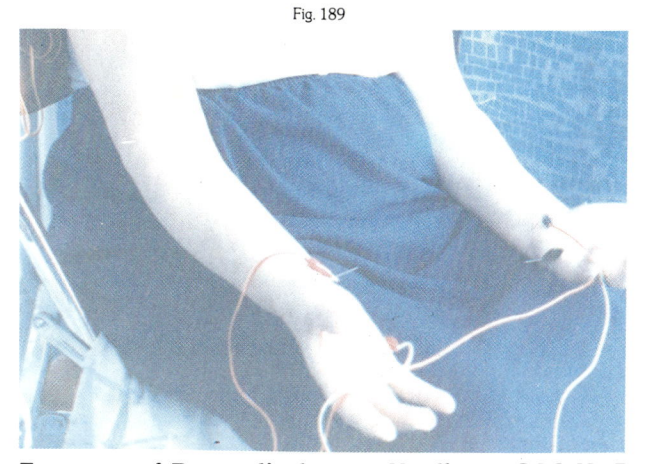

Fig. 189

Treatment of Raynaud's disease. Needles at S.I.2 Ht 7. Electro-stimulation.

MISCELLANEOUS FACTS & TREATMENTS

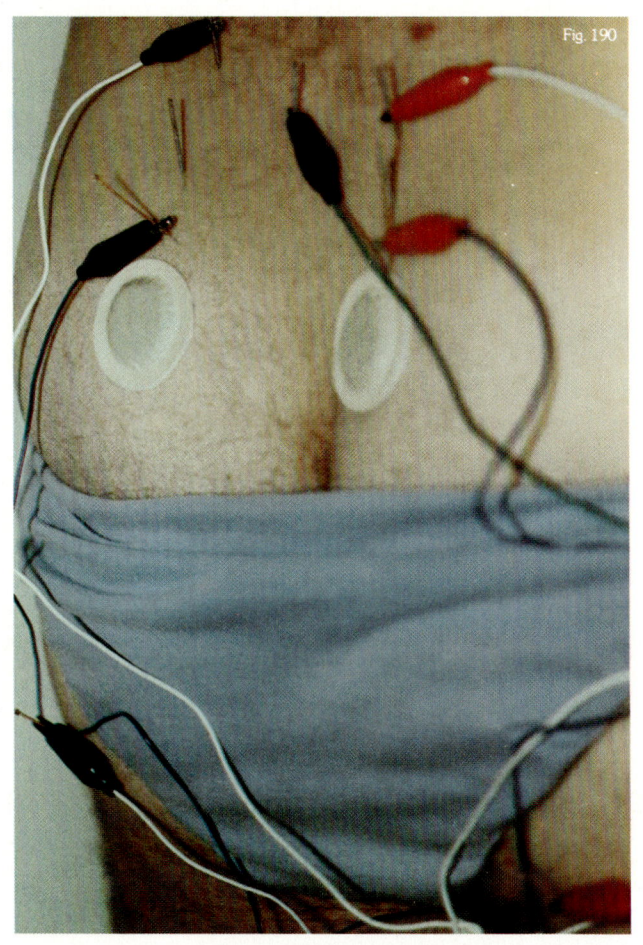

Fig. 190

Marukyu-Ban used for backache with needles.

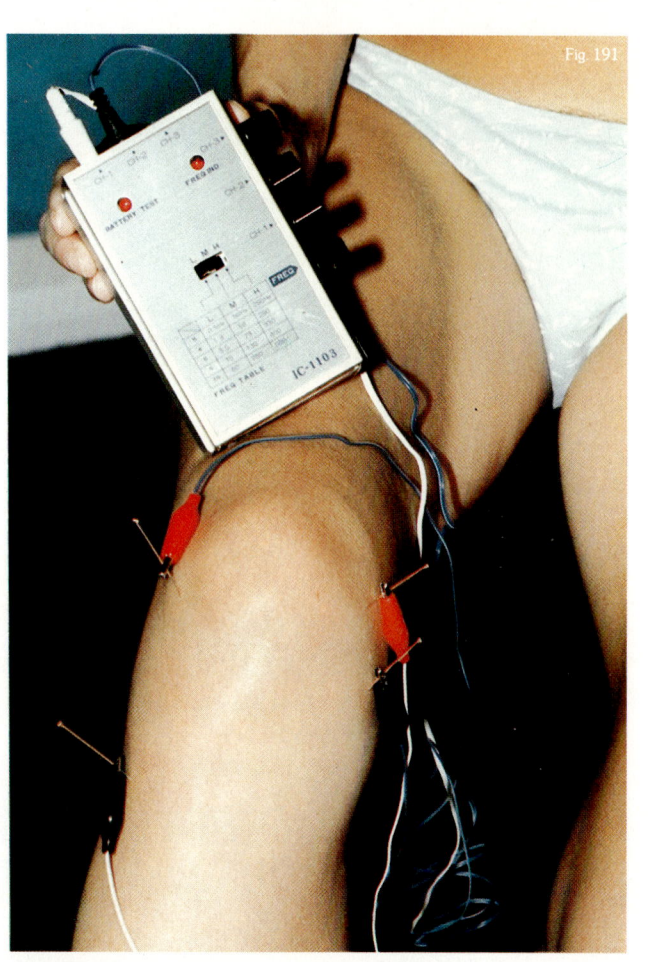

Fig. 191

Treatment of arthritis of the knee. Points as shown IC-1103 was used for electro-acupuncture.

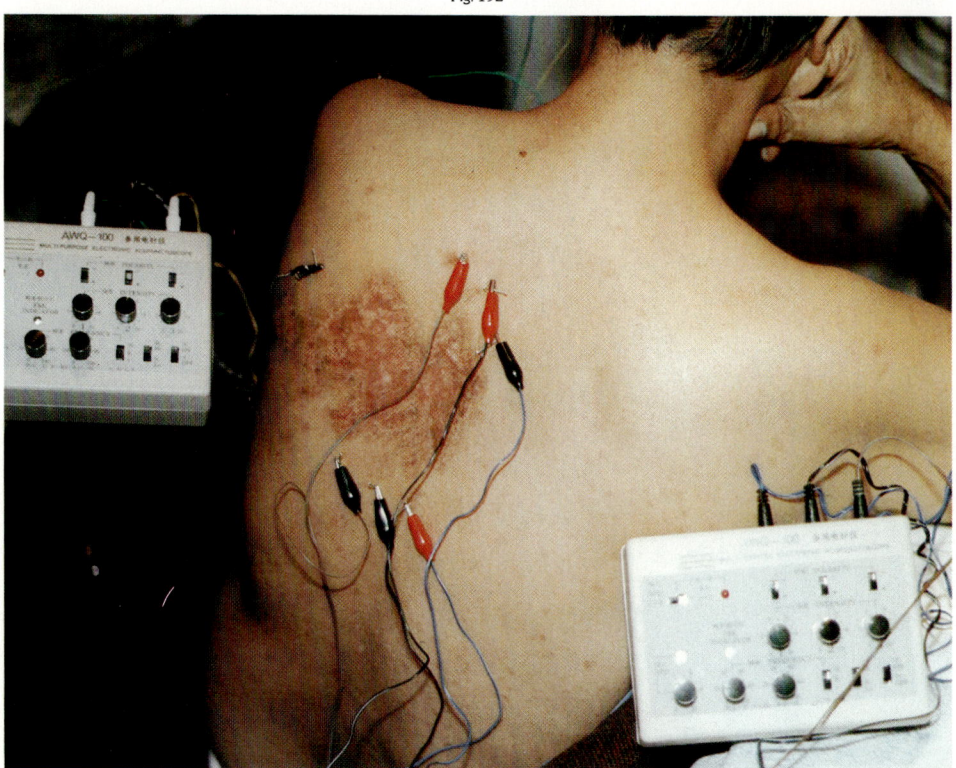

Fig. 192

Treatment of post herpatic neuralgia. Herpes zoster about 2 years ago but still was having pain. L 6th and 7th spinal nerves involved.

Treated with points above and below scar Bl_{12} Bl_{18} GV_8 SI_{11} Bl_{36} Bl_{42} GV_{10}
Electro-acupuncture WQ100.

Starting an Acupuncture Clinic

1. Needles - (a) Body Acupuncture ½inch to 6 inches
   (b) Semi-permanent needles for Ear Acupuncture
   (c) Forceps

2. Models and Charts

3. Anti-Tobacco plastic for 10 Needle Technique of Nogier

4. Moxa Rolls and Extinguisher, Moxa Wool, Mini Moxa

5. Seven Star Needle with electrical connection plug to Acupunctoscope

6. WQ-100 Multipurpose Electronic Acupunctoscope with reverse polarity, Acupuncture point detector. Also has 2 frequency controls F1, F2 for dense-disperse current, continuous current, Intermittent current. Multiplication Factor to 10. Frequencies - 1 to 1,000 Hertz. or IC-1107 Electro-Acupunctoscope

7. Diascope

8. Marukyu-Ban Thermal Plaster

9. Laser Machines
   Theralaser
   Unilaser - Infra-Red visible
   Helium Neon - Gumen Laser

STARTING AN ACUPUNCTURE CLINIC

THE FOLLOWING EQUIPMENT AND APPARATUS ARE ESSENTIAL FOR PRACTISING ACUPUNCTURE

1. Needles: ½", 1". 1½", 2", 3" to 6" Gauge 36 and metals — steel, gold, silver, molybdenum for body and ear acupuncture, semi-permanent needles — gold, steel and stilver for ear acupuncture.
2. Models and charts.
3. Moxa rolls, wool, mini-moxa and Marukyu-Ban for THERMAL THERAPY and Moxa extinguisher.
4. Seven star needle as shown in Fig. 200.
5. Anti-tobacco plastic for 10 needle technique of Nogier.
6. Forceps for insertion of semi-permanent needles.
7. Steriliser may be needed since the present day trend is to use disposable needles, this is not essential.
8. Medi swabs.
9. Comfortable couch is essential.
10. Acupuncture stimulators: WQ-100 multiple purpose electronic acupunctoscope with reversal of polarity and point detector and 2 frequency control is the BEST stimulator available. It also has a point finder and 3 outputs for 6 points.
11. THE DIASCOPE — differential detector and stimulator of auricular therapy and acupuncture points.
12. LASER APPARATUS
    1) Uni-laser
    2) Theralaser
    3) Gumem, He-neon laser are all preferred by the Author.

Fig. 193

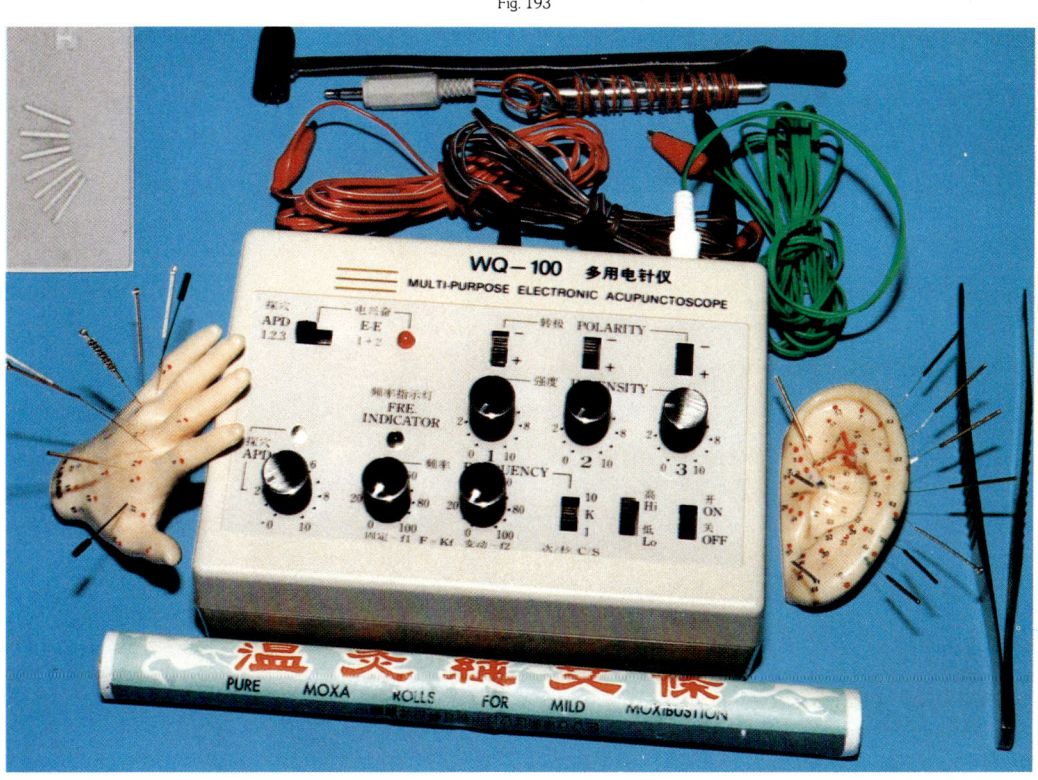

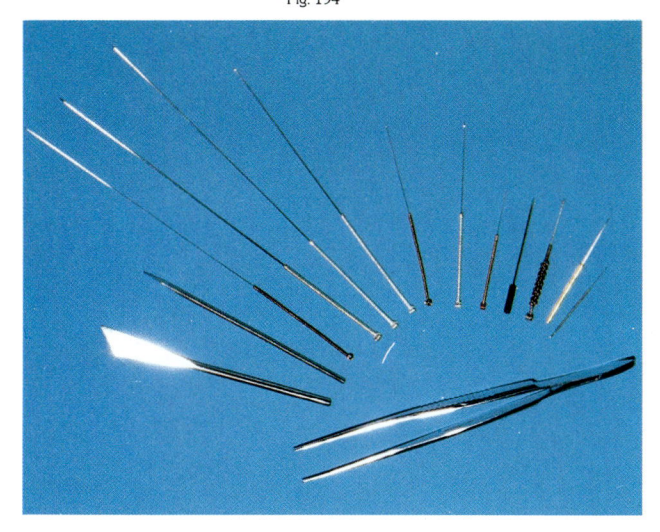

Fig. 194

Fig. 195

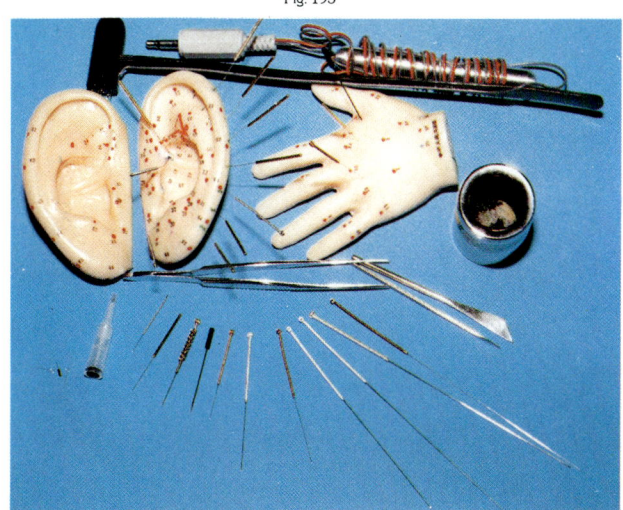

STARTING AN ACUPUNCTURE CLINIC

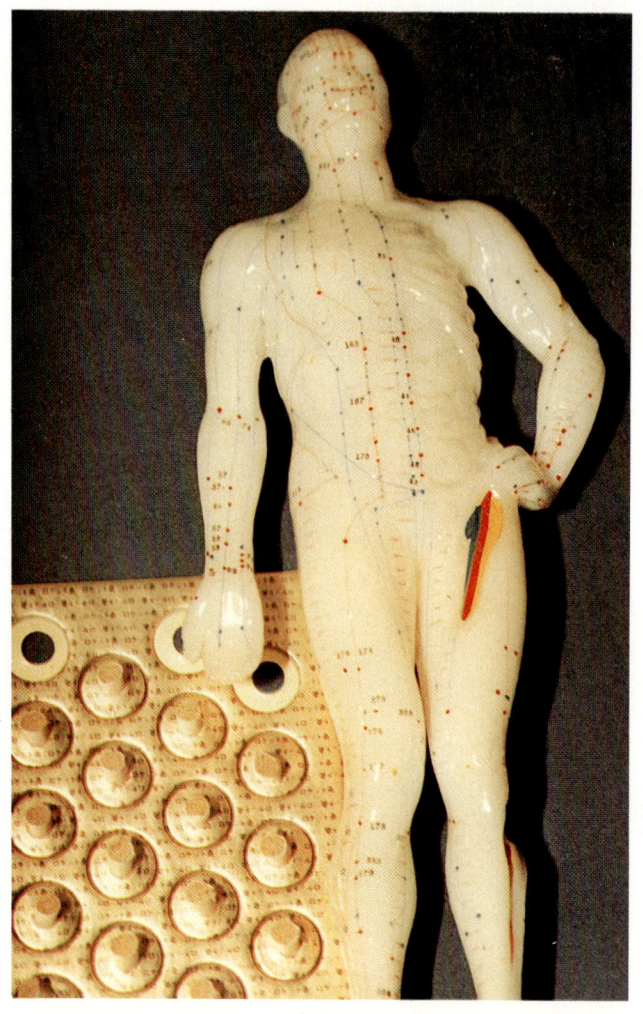

Fig. 196

Fig. 197

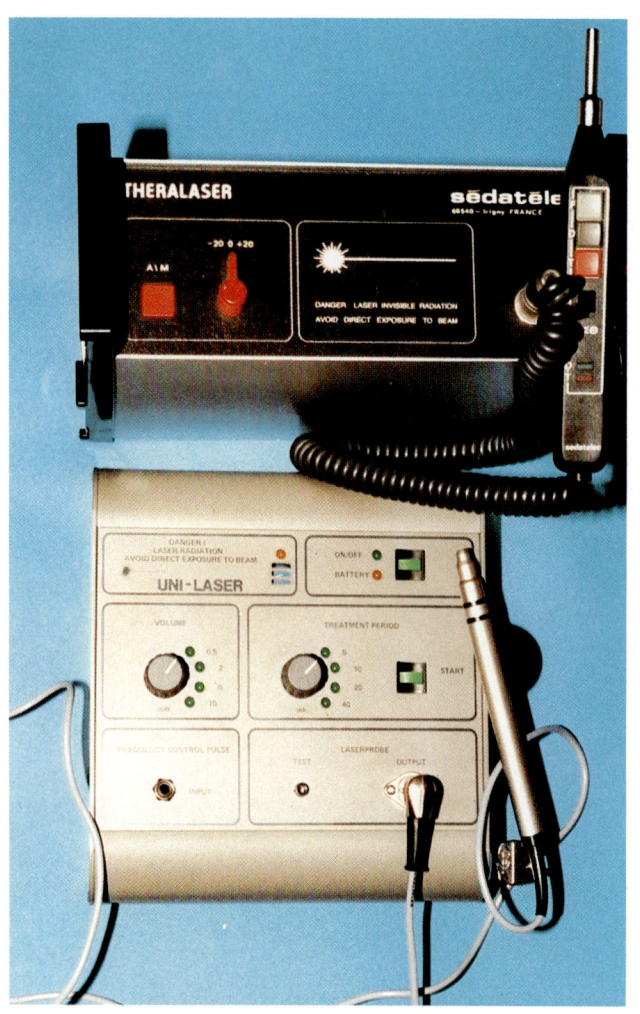

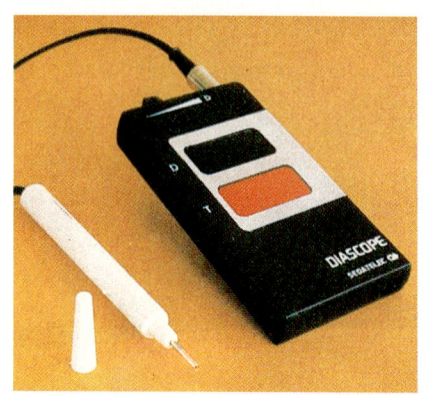

Fig. 198

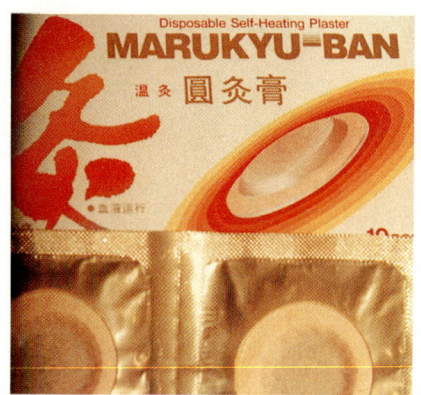

Fig. 199

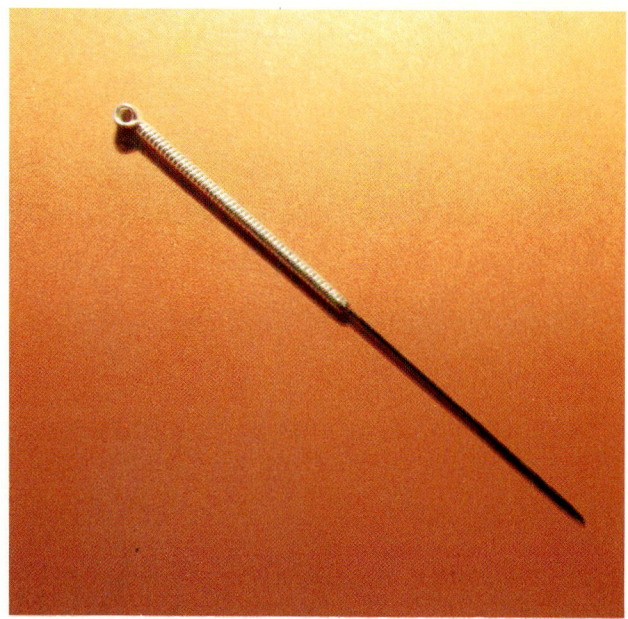

Fig. 200

Treatment of Heroin and Cocaine addiction, Chronic Alcoholism and Benzodiazepine Withdrawal

23

TREATMENT OF HEROIN, COCAINE ADDICTION AND CHRONIC ALCOHOLISM.

ACUPUNCTURE TREATMENT, has been found useful in the treatment of Heroin, Cocaine additiction and in Chronic Alcoholism and in the treatment of other habit forming drugs. In the latter group fewer sessions will be necessary.

In 1680 the English physician, Thomas Sydenham, wrote:

"Among the remedies which it has pleased Almighty God to give man to relieve his sufferings, none is so universal and so efficacious as opium." Over the intervening centuries the admiration of the medical community for the pain-relieving effects of opium and its derivatives has been tempered by an awareness of their toxicity and addictiveness. This awareness, together with the lack of any other known class of drugs that exert the powerful analgesic action of opiates, stimulated an intensive search for synthetic opiates with the good properties of morphine and without the bad ones. More recently natural morphine-like substances have been found in the brain. These substances promise to open new avenues to an understanding of precisely where in the body opiates act, how they do so and why they are addictive.

Drugs, hormones and neurotransmitters (chemicals released by nerve endings that modulate the firing of other nerve cells or neurones) all produce highly selective effects at very low concentration. It is usually assumed that they act at a specific receptor site consisting of large molecules and located on the external surface of cells in the target organs. For the opiate-like morphines, endorphins and enchephalin, a variety of evidence supports the receptor concept.

When acupuncture is used, two substances could be produced from the brain, spinal cord and pituitary gland. It has recently become known that electrical stimulation of the brain increases endorphin production which results in a higher endorphin level in the cerebrospinal fluid withdrawn from the lumbar region. Tests are being made to determine whether there is an increased production of endogenous opiates following percutaneous cervical cordotomy and the pituitary injection of alcohol when these procedures relieve pain.

It is abvious that endogenous opiate exists. Hughes et al. (1975) found two related pentapeptides — methionine enkephalin and leucine enkephalin — with activity at these sites. These substances have chains short enough to synthesise and it was shown that they have the same opiate activity and side effects as morphine.

They have a very short duration of action, being broken down very rapidly, while their opiate action is antagonized by naloxone. By immunoflourescent technique, Elde et al. (1976) showed that enkephalinergic axons existed in the c.n.s. at the opiate binding sites mentioned previously and they were also found in plexuses in the gut. It would appear that from this and other evidence that the enkephalins are neurotransmitter substances. These axons associated with these substances are very short except in the striatum.

Methionine enkephalin is formed by the breakdown of pituitary Beta-lipotropin together with another substance known as the C-fragment (now called Beta-endorphin) which is a much larger fragment of B-lipotropin.

A series of related substances have now been isolated which have opiate agonist activity. The endorphins have longer chains than the enkephalins with Beta-endorphin consisting of thirty-one amino-acids. It is present in the hypothalamus, the thalamus and other areas but not in the spinal cord. Enkephalin is rapidly destroyed. In fact, it is destroyed as rapidly as acetylcholine and because of this is ineffective when injected into the ventricles of the brain. Endorphin, on the contrary, is not so rapidly destroyed and is potent when injected into the ventricles.

There is no doubt that the mammalian brain contains peptides, the enkephalins and endorphins, which have, as stated earlier, pharmacological properties similar to those of morphine. Evidence for anatomical discrete pathway has emerged from the demonstrations that electrical stimulation via implanted electrodes of the periventricular and periaqueductual grey matter of man can substantially alleviate otherwise intractable pain.

When acupuncture, specially electro acupuncture is used, there is no doubt that these substances are released which is the possible means there is alleviation of pain.

It is also interesting to note that when continuous low frequency impulses are used, chemical that is released is endorphin. If naloxone, which reverses the effect of morphine, is injected to a patient who had had low freqency electro acupuncture, the effect of the endorphin is reversed by naloxone.

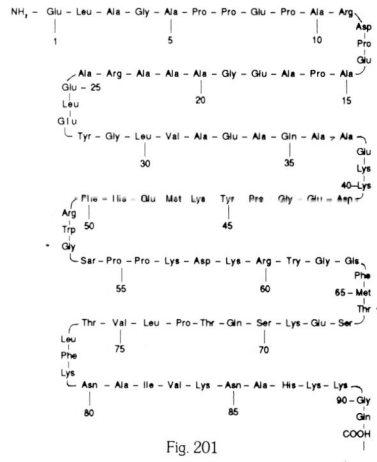

Fig. 201

The structure of beta-lipotropin incorporates several opioid peptides.

Peptide	Amino acid sequence
methionine-enkephalin	61 - 65
alpha-endorphin	61 - 76
gamma-endorphin	61 - 77
beta-endorphin	61 - 91

Ala	Alanine	Gly	Glycine	Phe	Phenylalanine
Arg	Arginine	Ile	Isoleucine	Pro	Proline
Asn	Asparagine	His	Histidine	Ser	Serine
Asp	Aspartic acid	Leu	Leucine	Thr	Threonine
Gln	Glutamine	Lys	Lysine	Trp	Tryptophan
Glu	Glutamic acid	Met	Methionine	Tyr	Tyrosine
				Val	Valine

Beta-Lipotropin, a pituitary peptide hormone 91 amino acids along, has amino acid sequences with several distinct physiological functions. The peptide chain as a whole induces the metabolism of fat, as does the segment termed gamma-lipotropin (amino acid units 1 through 58). The sequence 41 through 58 is that of the hormone beta-melanotropin, which plays a role in skin pigmentation. The sequence 61 through 91 is that of beta-endorphin, a pituitary peptide that has analgesic effects when it is injected intravenously or is injected directly into the brain. A second pituitary peptide, designated alpha-endorphin (61 through 76), has similar but less potent effects. The beta-lipotropin sequence 61 through 65 is identical with that of methionine-enkephalin, a morphine like peptide found in the brain, the spinal cord and the intestines. The relation between the opiate like peptides and the beta-lipotropin is not known.

DRUGS AND ALCOHOLISM

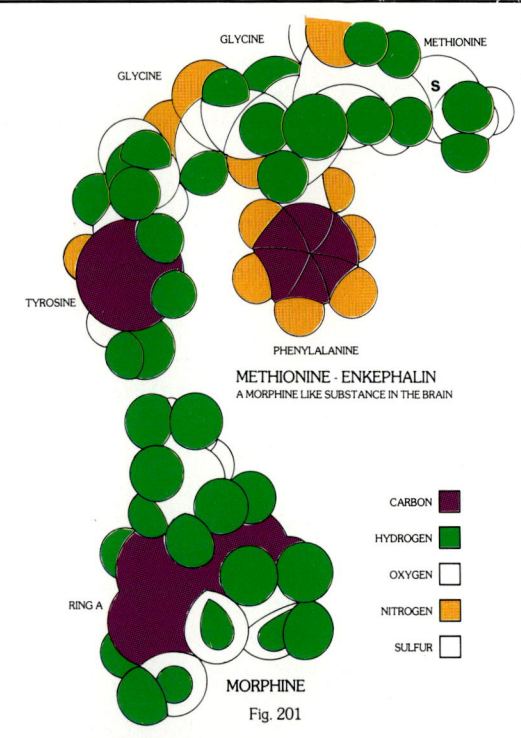

SPACE FILLING MOLECULAR MODELS of morphine (bottom) and methionine-enkephalin (top), a morphinelike substance in the brain, have some structural features in common. The benzene ring A of morphine that bears a hydroxyl group is in precisely the same orientation as the benzene ring of the amino acid tyrosine at one end of the enkephalin peptide chain, suggesting that this group binds to the opiate receptor in both cases. The second ring on the enkephalin molecule is that of the amino acid phenylalanine, and it appears to interact with the agonist conformation of the opiate receptor in much the same way that the benzene ring F of potent opiate agonist of are.

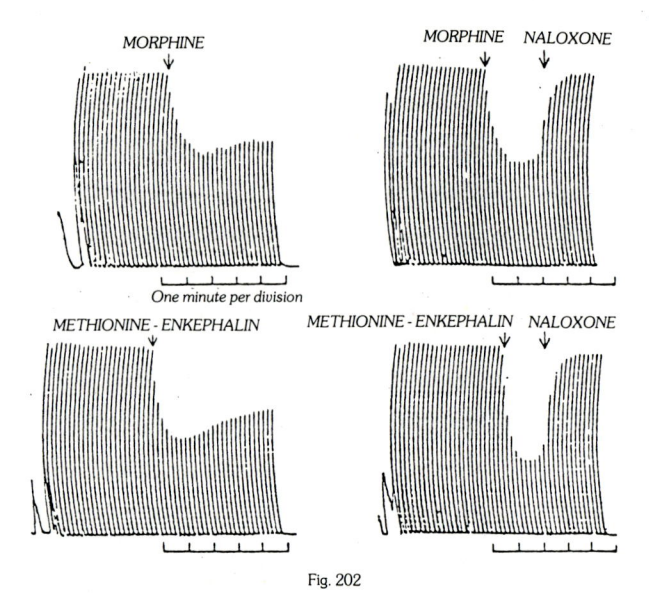

Fig. 201

Fig. 202

ENKEPHALIN MIMICS MORPHINE, inhibiting the electrically induced contractions of the guinea-pig intestine, in these polygraph readings
The inhibition of cokephalin, like that of morphine, is blocked by the antagonist naloxone. Similarity in the effects of the two compounds suggests that they act at same recepior.

It is interesting to note that if high frequency impulse is used in electro acupuncture enkephalin is released—methionine enkephalin is released and this is not reversed by naloxone but is reversed by 5HT which is 5 Hydroxy tryptamine which is serotonin.

Recently, a team at St. Bartholomews Hospital in London, has confirmed that the brain's own pain killing molecules, endorphin and enkephalin are released in people who have had acupuncture. It has been found that the treatment do cause increases in levels of the natural pain killers. The researchers studies also support another suspicion about the two classes of molecules: that they have different origins and actions.

Several other scientists have already forged links between acupuncture and some natural painkilling factor. Transferring cerebrospinal fluid (which surrounds the brain and the nerves in the spinal cord) from an animal that had acupuncture to one that has not will also transfer the painkilling effect, previous studies have shown. Furthermore, the inhibitor naloxone, which counters the effects of natural painkillers and of analgesic drugs also nullifies the effects of acupuncture.

In 1980 Dr. Vicky Clement Jones and her colleagues reported that heroin addicts having acupuncture treatment for their withdrawal symptoms had an increase in enkephalin levels in their cerebrospinal fluid after acupuncture. There was no increase of endorphin in these people, nor was there an increase in either molecule in the painfree patients who donated c.s.f. samples as controls.

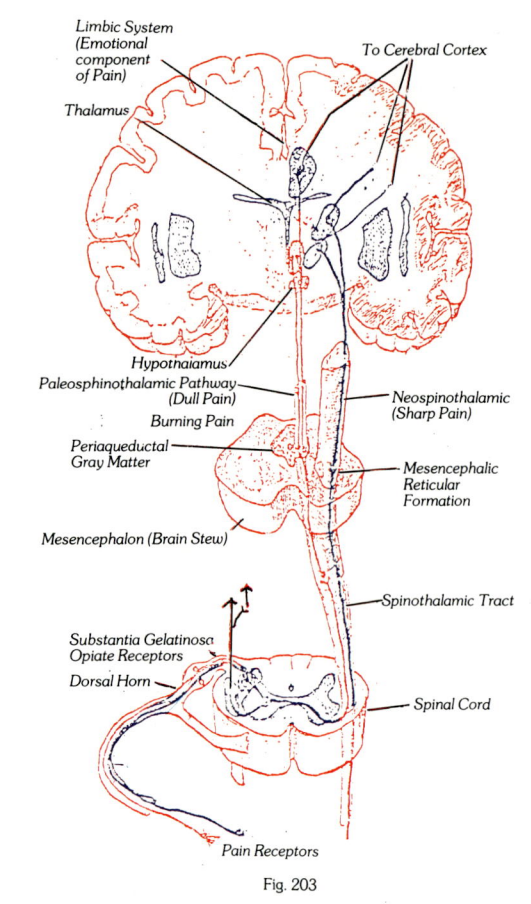

Fig. 203

Pain pathways carrying information from the periphery of the nervous system in the brain are separated into two types, the laterally localised pain and the medially localised paleospinothalamic pathway that transmits less localised burning pain. Burning pain is best relieved by opiates and the opiate receptors are found to be concentrated in the substantia gelatinosa and in the central thalamus.

Both Endogenous Opiates Endorphin and Encephalin are similar to Heroin but the Endogenous Opiates are more potent than Heroin or Diamorphine. Endorphins chemical structure is closer to Heroin, therefore if in Acupuncture treatment the brain spinal cord and the Pituitary Gland are made to release Encephalins better results could be achieved in the treatment of Heroin addiction. This can be done by setting needles at certain points both in the body and the ear (Auricular therapy) and stimulating the needle at high frequency (80 to 100 Hertz.) per second.

Heroin detoxification is difficult and about 8-12 sessions will be required in resistent cases.

In Western Medicine Methodone is used initially followed by Clonidine, Lomotil, Diazepam and in some cases a hypnotic such as Temazepam is used.

In this section only the acupuncture treatment will be given

DRUGS AND ALCOHOLISM

Acupuncture treatment of Heroin addiction and Chronic Alcoholism and Benzodiazepine Withdrawal. (Detoxification Programme)

A. BODY ACUPUNCTURE POINTS: Nervous Tension points, namely—
   G.V.20 and the 4 points 1 inch in front, behind and 1 inch lateral to G.V.20 on the right and left sides (refered as SHIN-SHEN-SHONG). These points are in the scalp.
   2. Conception vessel 17.
   3. In the upper limb Co4 Co11 Co15 bilaterally.
   4. Three Heater 16 apex of mastoid process bilaterally.
   5. In the lower limb Li3 Sp6 St36 bilaterally.

B. AURICULAR POINTS: Use the points used for the formula 10 needle technique of Paul Nogier. Use both ears and the needles are inserted with the anti-tobacco plastic the highest point being Darwin's point in the Darwin's tubercle.

   In addition use SHENMEN, JEROME and the ANTI-TRAGUS.

C. NEEDLES USED: Steel needles or silver needles are used for body points and gold for auricular points, but steel needles may be used if gold needles are not available.

D. Stimulation of needles with electronic acupunctuscope is essential with a frequency of 80 to 100 hertz.

E. Duration of treatment for a minimum of 40 minutes.

F. Number of sessions 8 - 12. Treatment at least two or three times a week.

G. Booster sessions may be required depending on response to therapy.

H. CONNECTION OF ELECTRODES: G.V.20 to C.V.17, Co4 to Co4, T.H.16 to T.H.16. All other points on the scalp, Li3 to Li3, Sp6 to Sp6, St36 to St36.
   Ear points Darwin's point of right ear to Darwin's point of left ear.
   Lowest point of on rim, i.e. 7th needle to 7th needle on the other ear, Anti-Aggression of right ear to Anti-Aggression of left ear.
   Shenmen of right ear to Shenmen of left ear.

For Auricular Points - place anti-tobacco protractor on ear, the highest slot is at Darwin's Tubercle. Use 10 needles, all same metals - gold (preferred) steel or silver - Fig. A

Fig. 204

Fig. 205

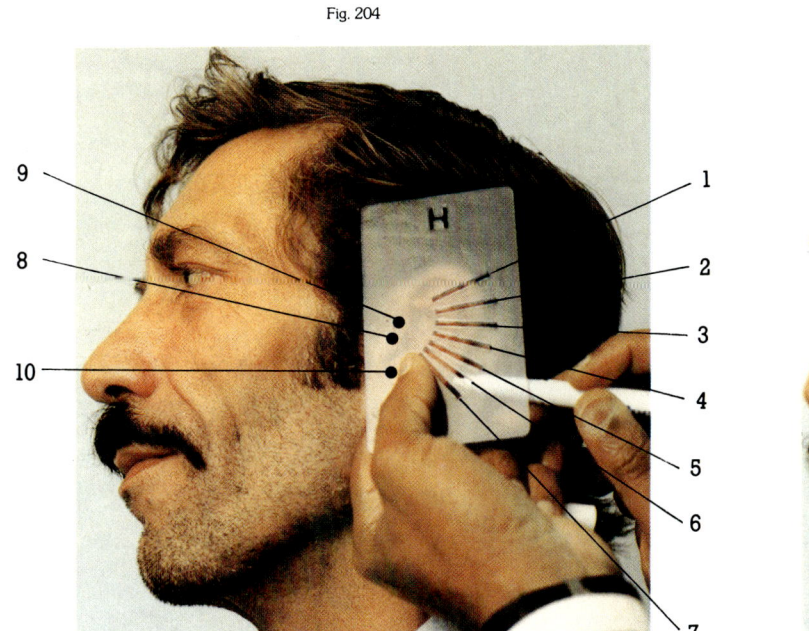

Figure A

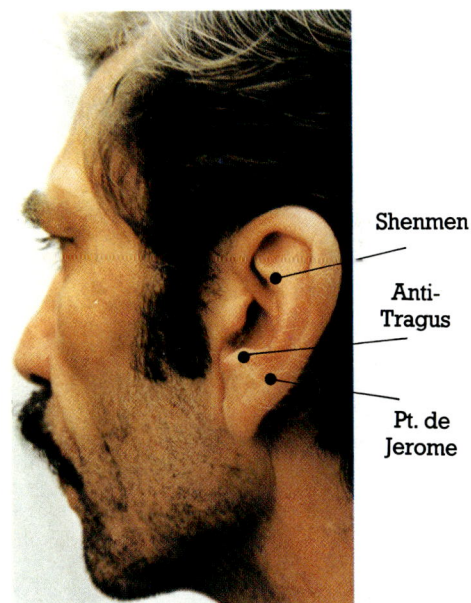

Figure B

10 half inch needles inserted. Connect needle 1 R. ear to needle 1 L. Ear, Connect needle 7 R. ear to needle 7 L. ear for stimulation.

DRUGS AND ALCOHOLISM

The people in these photgraphs are models and are not Drug Addicts or Alcoholics

Fig. 208

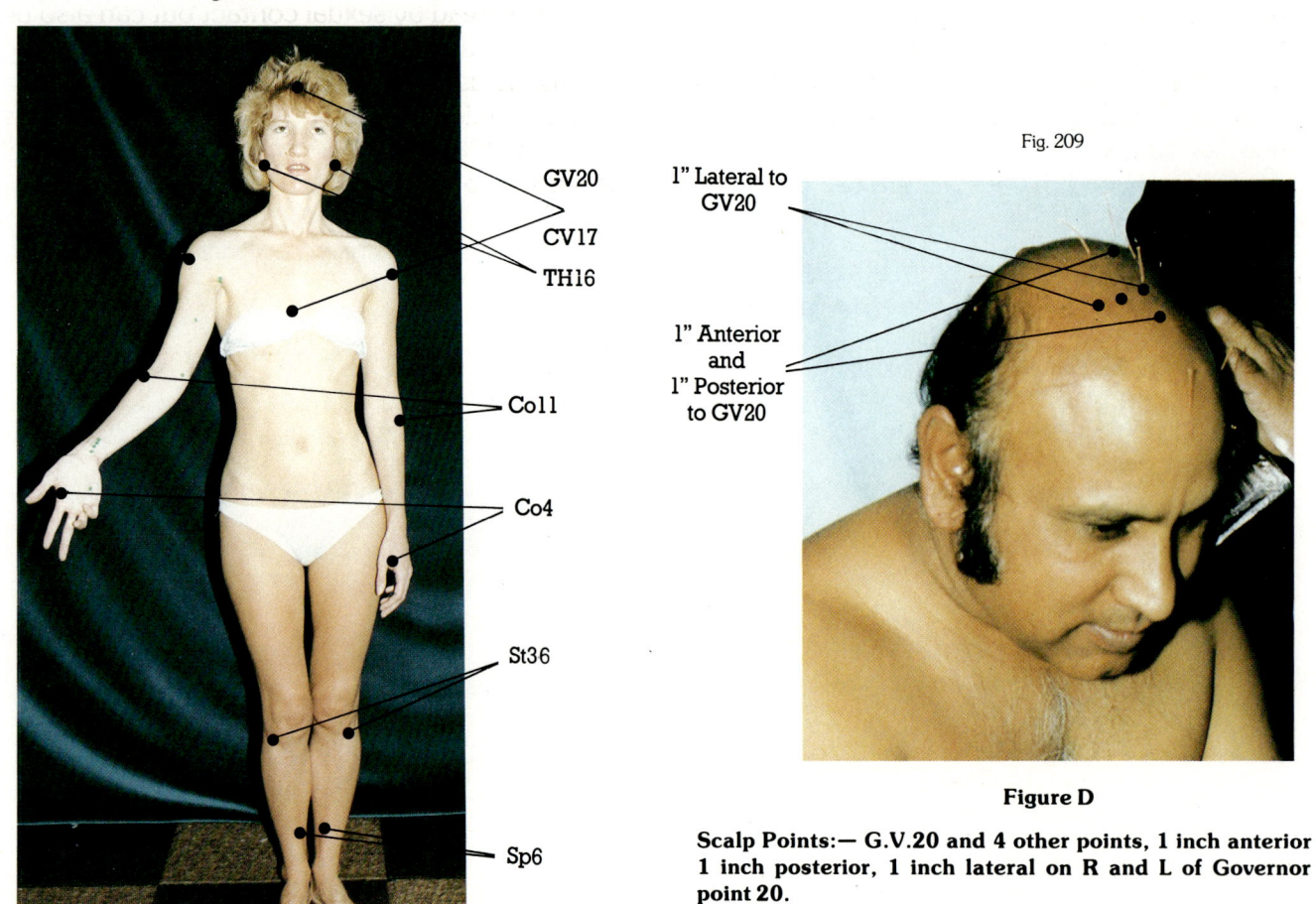

- GV20
- CV17
- TH16
- Co11
- Co4
- St36
- Sp6
- Li3

Figure C

Body points and their connections are shown in Fig. C

Fig. 209

- 1" Lateral to GV20
- 1" Anterior and 1" Posterior to GV20

Figure D

Scalp Points:— G.V.20 and 4 other points, 1 inch anterior 1 inch posterior, 1 inch lateral on R and L of Governor point 20.

Figures E. and F. - on the rim of Helix are shown the 7 points obtained using anti-tobacco plastic. Connect points 1 and 7 and stimulate for 40 mins.

Fig. 210

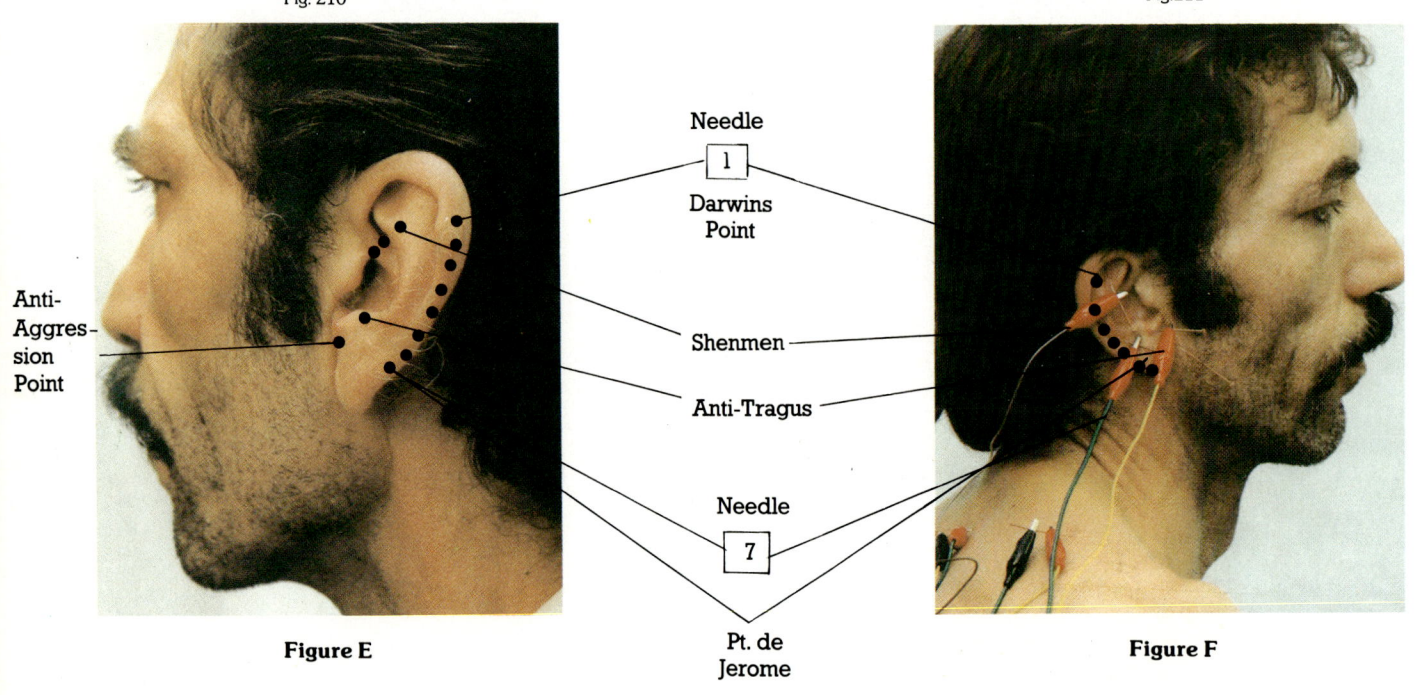

Anti-Aggression Point

- Needle 1
- Darwins Point
- Shenmen
- Anti-Tragus
- Needle 7
- Pt. de Jerome

Figure E

Fig. 211

Figure F

DRUGS AND ALCOHOLISM

THE USE OF DISPOSABLE ACUPUNCTURE NEEDLES

The HIV virus is known to be the cause of the Acquired Immune Deficiency Syndrome (AIDS) and of AIDS-related complex (ARC). The virus is predominantly spread by sexual contact but can also be spread by inoculation of infected body fluids, in particular by the sharing of needles amongst drug addicts. HIV infection is also known to be spread by the transfusion of infected blood and by the use of other blood products such as factor VIII. There is a theoretical risk that the use of acupuncture needles can spread the HIV virus. The spread of the hepatitis B virus by this method is well recognised. For this reason, the use of disposable needles is to be recommended.

PRE-STERILIZED DISPOSABLE ACUPUNCTURE NEEDLES

Fig. 212

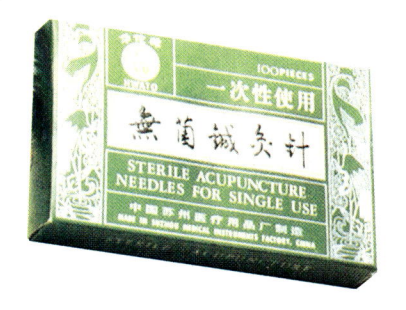

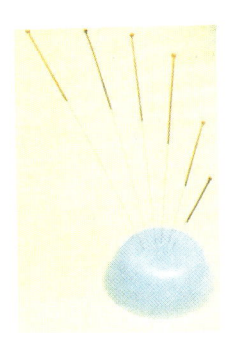

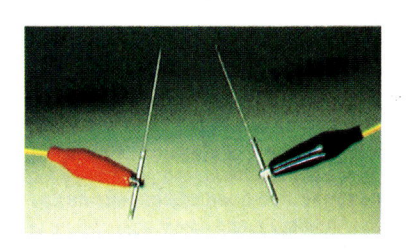

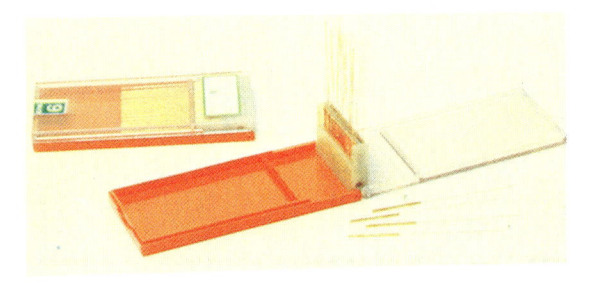

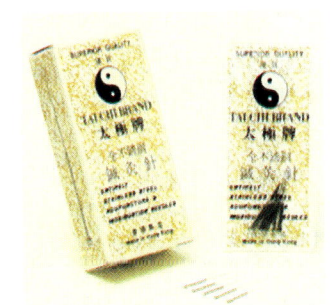

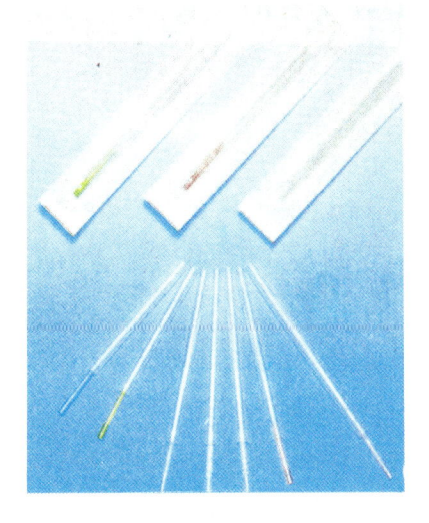

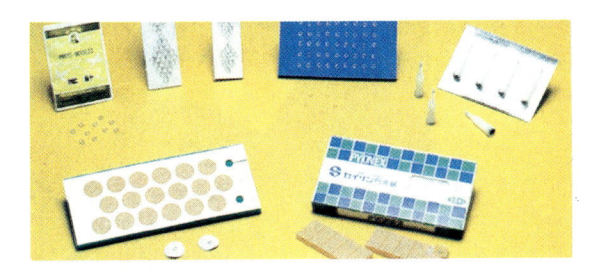

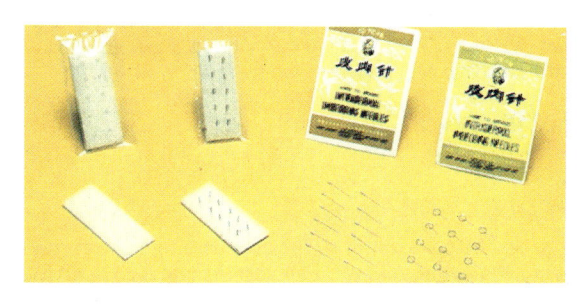

MARINA BRAND

ACUPUNCTURE NEEDLES

SUPERIOR QUALITY STAINLESS STEEL

MARINA ACADEMY **MARINA SUPPLIES**

30,32 LISMORE ROAD, SOUTH CROYDON CR2 7QA
ENGLAND. TEL: 01-680 0774

MARINA SUPPLIES

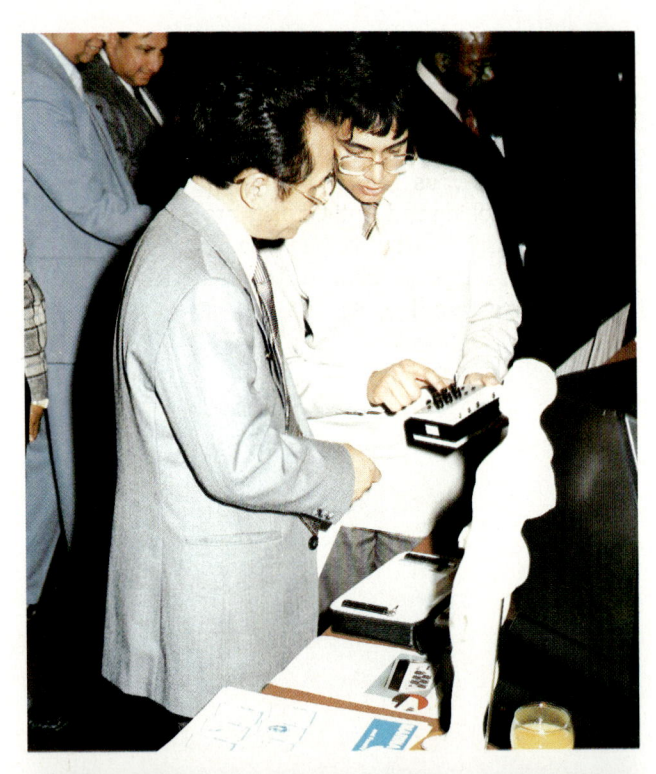

Dr. Karim Meeran explaining to one of the delegates at the Marina Supplies stall the workings of a WQ-100 electronic electro-acupunctoscope. IInd World Acupuncture Congress held in London, May 1986.

IInd International Acupuncture Congress May 1986. Marina Academy and Supplies International stall.

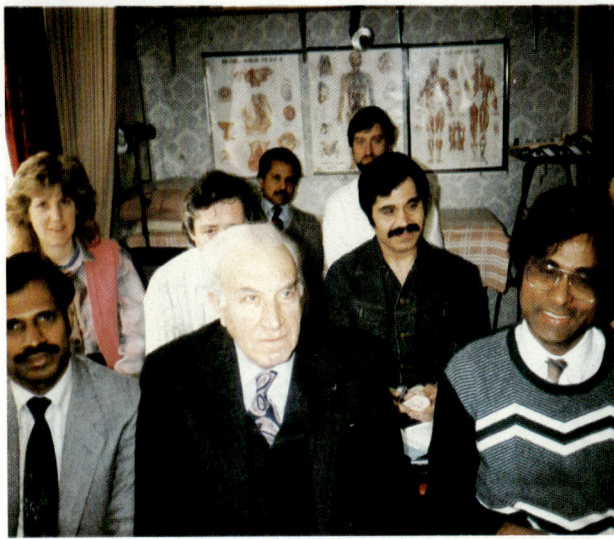

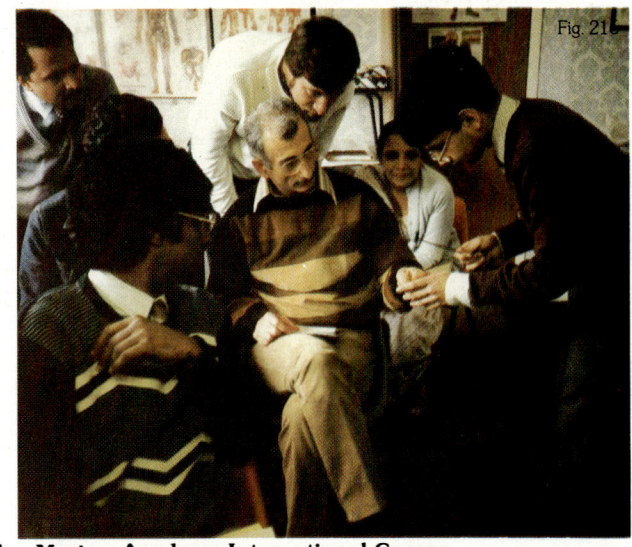

Doctors who attended the 55th Course of the Marina Academy International Course conducted regularly by the Academy.

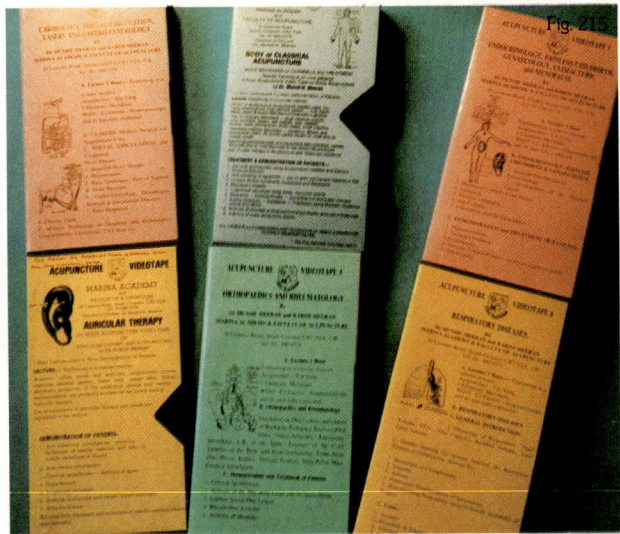

Acupuncture video tapes available from Marina Supplies International.

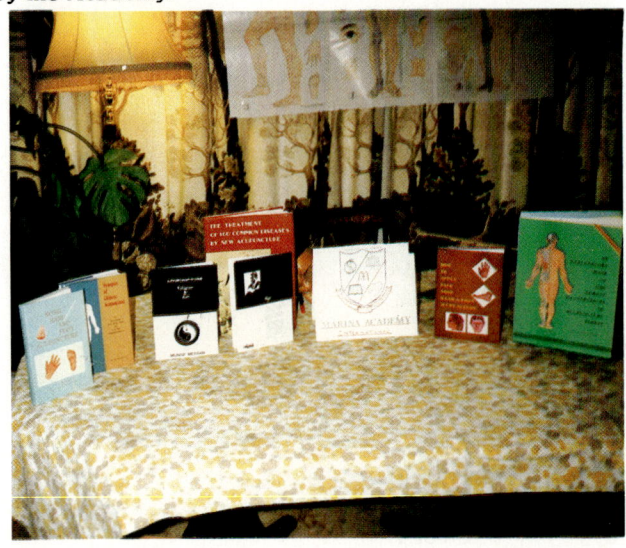

Books and equipment available from Marina Acadamy and Supplies International.

ACUPUNCTURE COURSES

Course in Acupuncture, Moxibustion, Electro-Acupuncture, Auriculotherapy and Laser Therapy in Acupuncture

1. What is Acupuncture?
2. Yin-Yang theory and five element system.
3. Theories of Acupuncture.
4. Acupuncture Points and Meridians in general.
5. Pulse Diagnosis and the Chinese Clock.
6. Techniques of Acupuncture and sterilisation of needles.

Meridians of Acupuncture

1. Colon
2. Lung
3. Spleen
4. Stomach
5. Heart
6. Pericardium
7. Small Intestine
7. Small Intestine
9. Gall Bladder
10. Liver
11. Bladder
12. Kidney
13. Conception (Ren)
14. Governor (Brain) Meridian

1. Moxibustion
2. Neuro-Chemical Transmitters
3. Endorphin-Encephalin theory.
4. Physiology of pain.
5. The Gate control theory of Melzack and Wall.
6. Prostaglandins and Anti-Prostaglandins.

AURICULAR-THERAPY (Ear Acupuncture)

1. Anatomy of the Ear.
2. Types of needle used in Ear Acupuncture.
3. Auricular points, their detection, Reflex Cartography of the Auricle, including zones on the medial surface of the Auricle.
4. Auricular Acupuncture for the treatment of disease.

ELECTRO ACUPUNCTURE

1. Principles and mode of application.
2. Demonstration of instruments used in Acupuncture.
3. Constant and Dense-Disperse Currents.
4. Method of connecting points when using Electro-Acupuncture.
5. Electro-Acupuncture Machines.

   Patient Demonstration.

Auricular Therapy (Ear Acupuncture)(Continued)

1. Cosmetic Acupuncture.
2. Projection of the Central Nervous system, endocrines, Autonomic Nervous system, Musculo-skeletal system, Thorax and Abdomen.
3. Formulae for Smoking, Obesity and Impotence, Frigidity, Phobias and Nervous Tension.
4. Meeran Technique for Press needle insertion into Auricle.
5. Combination of Auricular Therapy and Classical Acupuncture.

LASERS

1. Introduction.
2. Physics and Essential Physical Properties of a Laser Beam.
3. Effects of the Laser Beam on Tissue.
4. Lasers in Medicine, Surgery and Acupuncture.
5. Technique of Treatment using the Theralaser.
6. Points, Time and Modulation in Laser Therapy.
7. The Seven frequencies: A, B, C, D, E, F, G.

Treatment of Disease

1. General Principles.
2. General Aspects of Treatment.
3. Use of Nervous Tension Points.
4. Anti-smoking and Anti-Obesity programme.
5. Treatment of Arthritis, Migraine, Nervous-Tension, Hypertension, Backache, Trigeminal Neuralgia, Tinnitus, Vertigo, etc.
6. Treatment of Impotence, Frigidity and Sub-fertility.
7. Painless Childbirth.

Practical Demonstration on Patients

Practical demonstration will take place throughout the Course.

OTHER COURSES AVAILABLE

ANATOMY COURSE

Histology, Upper Limb, Lower Limb, Head and Neck Thorax, Abdomen, Pelvis, Nervous System

SURGERY COURSE

Structure - Function, Vascular Surgery, Neurosurgery, Endocrinology, Gastro-enterology, Chest & Heart Diseases Urology, Orthopaedics, Tumours

OBSTETRICS COURSE

Antenatal Care, Normal Pregnancy and Labour, Abnormal Labour, Toxaemia of Pregnancy, Twins and Hydramnios Breech, APH & PPH, Induction of Labour, Instrumental Delivery, Caesarean Section, Pre-maturity & Post-maturity, R.H. Factor, Ultrasound in Obstetrics - Scans

MEDICAL COURSE

Anatomy Physiology Embryology, Pathology, Body Fluids, Electrolytes, Lymphatics, Orthopaedics, Neurosurgery, Ailmentary System, Gastroenterlogy, Urology, Acute Abdomen, Tumours, Skin, Respiratory Diseases, Cardiology, E.C.G. X-ray, Obstetrics & Gynaecology, Pharmacology, Paediatrics, Tropical Diseases, Metabolic Diseases, Infectious Diseases

I: MEDICAL AND SURGERY COURSES

Courses in Anatomy, Surgery, Medicine, Paediatrics, Obstetrics and Gyneacology for postgraduate and medical students.

COURSES FOR:
P.L.A.B., M.B.B.S., L.R.C.P., M.R.C.S., D.R.C.O.G., F.R.C.S.(Gen.Surg), Parts I and II.

INDEX

A
acne: 83
acromegaly: 72
acth: 54; 97
acupuncture clinic: 123
acupuncture courses: 135
acupunctoscope: 15-16
addiction: 129
adrenal: 54
aids: 133
alcoholism: 129
alopecia: 84
anatomy of the breast: 98
ankle sprain: 72
anti-obesity: 77
anti-smoking: 77
anti- tobacco protractor: 15; 79; 132
antihelix: 51
anxiety: 93
aphasia: 115
aphonia: 115
arthritis of shoulder: 72
arthritis: 39; 71
assessment: 55
aum: 19
auriculotherapy: 47
autonomic nervous system: 52

B
back ache: 40; 65
bahui: 121
baldness: 84
bells palsy: 75-76
benzodiazepenes: 131
beta-lipotrophin: 129
bladder meridian: 28
blastocyst: 103
bone pain: 100
bones: 7
breast development: 97-100
bromocriptine: 104

C
calcitonin: 100
calcium: 100
carpal tunnel syndrome: 72
cephalo-pelvic disproportion: 88
cerebral hemisphere: 116
cervical spondylosis: 70
charts: 125
childbirth: 85
chinese monad: 1
clomiphene: 104
cocaine: 129
colon meridian: 23
conception: 103
conception meridian: 35
concha: 51
contractions: 87
corona technique: 45
cosmetic acupuncture: 83; 97
cranial meridians: 21
cranium: 7
cun: 19; 36

D
darwins point: 131
dermatology: 83
diagnosis: 57
diascope: 125
diencephalon: 53
disc lesion: 70
disposable needles: 133
dyspareunia: 105

E
ear acupuncture: 47-54
ear chart: 49
ear geometry: 53
earth: 1
eclampsia: 88
electro-acupuncture: 13-17
electro-acupuncture; advantages: 16
electrodes: 17
encephalin: 39; 129
endocrinology: 54; 95
endorphin: 39; 129
endoscopy: 57
episiotomy: 87
equipment: 125
extra-ordinary meridian: 1; 33

F
face: 75
fallopian tube: 103
fire: 1
five elements: 1
foot: 109
forceps delivery: 87
formula: 55
frigidity: 105

G
gall bladder meridian: 27
gastric area: 117
gate control theory: 37
golf elbow: 72
governor meridian: 35
growth hormone: 97

H
hand: 109
head: 115
headaches: 81
heart meridian: 24
helium-neon lasers: 44

INDEX

helix: 51
hepatitis B: 133
heroin: 129
herpes zoster: 121
hiv virus: 133
hydroxy tryptamine: 130
hypercalcaemia: 69; 97
hyperparathyroidism: 100
hypothalamus: 54

I
impotence: 105
infertility: 103
infra-red lasers: 44

J
joints: 8

K
kidney meridian: 29
ko cycle: 1

L
labour: 87
lactation: 97
laser mechanism: 43
laser therapy: 41
ligaments: 8
liver meridian: 29
lower limb: 61
lumbo-sacral disc: 40
lung meridian: 23

M
malignant hypercalcaemia: 97
mammary gland: 97
marina academy: 135
marukyu ban: 122
meeran's 12 needle technique: 100
meeran's laws: 36
meeran's technique for drug addiction: 131-132
melzack and wall: 37
menieres syndrome: 76
meridian: 1
mesencephalon: 53
metal: 1
migraine: 61
models: 125
morula: 103
motor area: 117
moxibustion: 15
muscles: 9

N
nail point: 21; 36
naloxone: 129
needles: 13-15; 125
nervous tension points: 93
neurology: 73
nogier: 50
nose: 109

O
obesity: 77
optic area: 117
ordinary meridian: 1;19
orthopaedics: 63
osteo arthritis: 71
oxytocin: 97

P
pacemaker: 17
pain: 59
pain pathway: 37
painless childbirth: 85-87
parasympathetic: 53
pericardium meridian: 24
peripheral vascular disease: 76
phobias: 93
pituitary: 54
placenta praevia: 88
pneumothorax free needle insertion: 83
post coital test: 104
pre-eclampsia: 88
progesterone: 97
prolactin: 97
prostaglandin: 39
psycho-somatics: 91

R
raynauds disease: 121
recti-linear stroking: 45
ren meridian: 35
rheumatoid arthritis: 71
rheumatology: 63
rotator cuff syndrome: 72

S
sarcoidosis: 100
scalp: 115
scaphoid fossa: 51
scars; removal of: 84
schizophrenia: 93
sciatica: 65; 70
sensory area: 117
serotonin: 130
shin-sheng-shong: 131
sinusitis: 81
skeletal system: 5
skull: 7
small intestine meridian: 26
smoking: 77
sperm antibodies: 103
sperm count: 104
spinal tumours: 68

INDEX

T
tamoxifen: 104
telencephalon: 52
ten needle technique: 79
tennis elbow: 72
tension: 93
theralaser: 43-44
thomas sydenham: 129
thoracic area: 117
three heater meridian: 30
thyroxine: 54; 97
tinnitus: 76
tragus: 51
triangular fossa: 51
trigeminal neuralgia: 75

U
unilaser: 44

V
vascular supply of the breast: 99
vertebral column tumours: 69
vertigo: 76
video tapes: 134

W
water: 1
wilfred perera; painless childbirth: 88
wood: 1
wq100 acupunctoscope: 15-16
wrinkles: 84

Y
yag laser: 44
yang: 1
yin: 1

Z
zero point of nogier: 49; 121
zygote: 103

MARINA ACADEMY

ACUPUNCTURE VIDEOTAPE

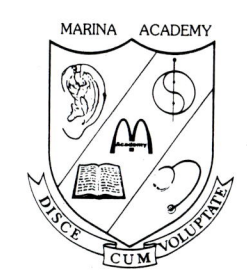

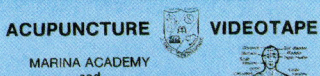

MARINA ACADEMY and FACULTY OF ACUPUNCTURE
30 Lismore Road,
South Croydon, CR2 7QA
Tel: 01-680 0774
Director of Studies:
Dr. Munsif H. Meeran

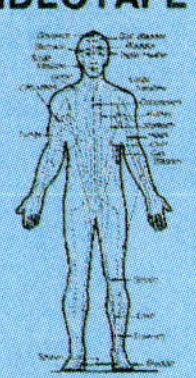

BODY or CLASSICAL ACUPUNCTURE

BODY MERIDIANS or CHANNELS and TREATMENT
Needle Technique on nine patients.
3 Hour Acupuncture Video Tape on Body Acupuncture
by Dr. Munsif H. Meeran

1½ Hour Lecture and 1½ Hour Demonstration of Patients.

Lecture: Explaining in a concise manner:

Origin of acupuncture, acupuncture needles used, Yin-Yang phenomenon, Five element system — Fire, Earth, Metal, Water & Wood, Meridians or Channels in general.
The 12 Ordinary Meridians — large intestine (colon), lung, stomach, spleen, gall bladder, liver, bladder, kidney, heart, pericardium, three heater, small intestine.
The Extra-ordinary Meridians — Governor (Brain) and Conception (Ren). All points clearly shown on chart and on human model.
Electro-Acupunctoscopes and equipment demonstrated, namely WQ-10B and IC 1103 and how to use electro-acupuncture.
Use of Laser therapy in Acupuncture and *Diascope explained.

TREATMENT & DEMONSTRATION OF PATIENTS:—
1. Cervical spondylosis using Acupuncture needles and Electro-Acupunctoscope.
2. Anti-smoking programme — use of semi-permanent needles in Ear.
3. Irritable Bowel Syndrome, Dyspepsia and Backache.
4. Raynaud's disease.
5. Trigeminal neuralgia using Body, Auricular points.
6. Backache — Osteoarthrosis — using Electro-and Laser therapy.
7. Kypho-Scoliosis — Backache — Treatment using Bladder, Governor points and Moxa.
*8. Arthritis of shoulder and carpal tunnel syndrome, also use of Diascope.
9. Arthritis of knee using body points.

ALL CASES FULLY DISCUSSED AND TECHNIQUE OF NEEDLE INSERTION CLEARLY DEMONSTRATED

* ON PAL/SECAM SYSTEM ONLY.

ACUPUNCTURE VIDEOTAPE 3

ORTHOPAEDICS AND RHEUMATOLOGY

By
Dr MUNSIF MEERAN and KARIM MEERAN
MARINA ACADEMY & FACULTY OF ACUPUNCTURE

30 Lismore Road, South Croydon CR2 7QA, UK.
Tel: 01 - 680 0774

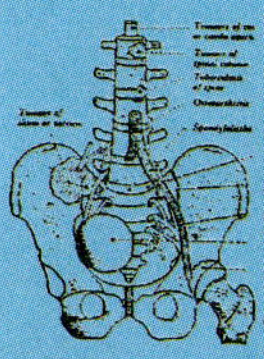

A. Lecture 1 Hour
Explaining in a concise manner
Acupuncture - Yin Yang.
5 Elements, Meridians.
WQ10 C2-Electro Acupunctoscope
and its uses fully explained.

B. Orthopaedics and Rheumatology.

Discussion on Disc Lesions and causes of Backache Prolapsed Intervertabral Discs, Osteo-Arthrosis, Ankylosing, Spondilitis, T.B. of the Spine, Tumours of the Cord, Tumours of the Bone and Bone secondaries, From Bronchus, Breast, Kidney, Thyroid, Prostate, Intra Pelvic Mass. Cervical Spondylosis.

C. Demonstration and Treatment of Patients
1. Cervical Spondylosis
2. Arthritis of the Hip using Laser and its applications.
3. Lumbar Sacral Disc Lesion.
4. Rheumatoid Arthritis.
5. Arthritis of Shoulder.

ACUPUNCTURE VIDEOTAPE 6

RESPIRATORY DISEASES.

BY
Dr MUNSIF MEERAN and KARIM MEERAN
MARINA ACADEMY & FACULTY OF ACUPUNCTURE

30 Lismore Road, South Croydon CR2 7QA, UK.
Tel: 01 - 680 0774

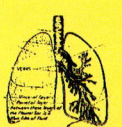

A. Lecture 1 Hour:— Explaining in a concise manner
Acupuncture - Yin Yang.
5 Elements, Meridians.
WQ10 C2-Electro Acupunctoscope
and its uses fully explained.

B. RESPIRATORY DISEASES
1. GENERAL INTRODUTION

1. Physiology of Respiration - Tidal Volume, FEV_1, Vital Capacity, Residual Volume, Total Lung Volume.

2. Graphs showing (a) normal function (b) Restrictive Airways (c) Obstructive Airways Etc.

1. Bronchitis and Emphysema
2. Sinusitis
3. Asthma
4. Pulmonary Manifestations of Sarcoidosis.
5. Anti-Smoking Programme using 10 Needle Technique of Nogier.

C. Cases:-
1. Asthma
2. Bronchitis & Emphysema.
3. Allergies.
4. 10 Needle Technique of Nogier.

ACUPUNCTURE VIDEOTAPE

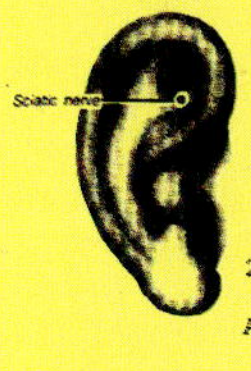

MARINA ACADEMY and FACULTY OF ACUPUNCTURE
30 Lismore Road, South Croydon, CR2 7QA
Tel: 01-680 0774
Director of Studies: Dr Munsif H. Meeran

AURICULAR THERAPY

2½ HOUR ACUPUNCTURE VIDEO TAPE
ON
AURICULAR THERAPY (EAR ACUPUNCTURE)
by DR MUNSIF MEERAN

1 Hour Lecture and 1½ Hour Demonstration of Patients.

LECTURE:— Explaining in a concise manner:

Anatomy, reflex zones and auricular acupuncture points, muscular skeletal system, lower limb, upper limb, thorax, abdomen, projection of the endocrine glands and central nervous system, ear geometry and special ear points used in auricular therapy.

Use of equipment in auricular therapy and needs are explained in the lecture.

DEMONSTRATION OF PATIENTS:
1. Anti-smoking programme showing technique of needle insertion and also 10 needle technique of Nogier.
2. Anti-obesity programme
3. Cervical spondylosis — Arthritis of spine.
4. Hypertension.
5. Trigeminal neuralgia.
6. Arthritis of shoulder and carpal tunnel syndrome.
7. Arthritis of knee.

All cases fully discussed and technique of needle insertion clearly demonstrated.

ACUPUNCTURE VIDEOTAPE 5

ENDOCRINOLOGY, PAINLESS CHILDBIRTH, GYNAECOLOGY, CLIMACTERIC and MENOPAUSE

BY
Dr MUNSIF MEERAN and KARIM MEERAN
MARINA ACADEMY & FACULTY OF ACUPUNCTURE

30 Lismore Road, South Croydon CR2 7QA, UK.
Tel: 01 - 680 0774

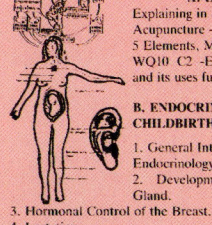

A. Lecture 1 Hour
Explaining in a concise manner
Acupuncture - Yin Yang.
5 Elements, Meridians.
WQ10 C2 -Electro Acupunctoscope
and its uses fully explained.

B. ENDOCRINOLOGY, PAINLESS CHILDBIRTH & GYNAECOLOGY.

1. General Introduction to Endocrinology.
2. Development of the Pituitary Gland.
3. Hormonal Control of the Breast.
4. Lactation.
5. Painless Childbirth.
6. Sub-Fertility.
7. Climacteric and the Menopause.

C. DEMONSTRATION and TREATMENT OF PATIENTS.
1. Hypothyroidism
2. Painless Childbirth.
3. Dyspareunia.
4. Nervous Tension Points. - shown as a general guide.
5. Sub-Fertility.

ACUPUNCTURE VIDEOTAPE 4

NEUROLOGY AND PSYCHIATRY

By
Dr MUNSIF MEERAN and KARIM MEERAN
MARINA ACADEMY & FACULTY OF ACUPUNCTURE

30 Lismore Road, South Croydon CR2 7QA, UK.
Tel: 01 - 680 0774

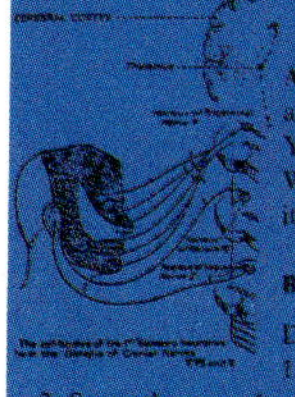

A. LECTURE 1 Hour:— Explaining in a concise manner Acupuncture - Yin-Yang. 5 Elements, Meridians WQ10 C2-Electro- Acupunctoscope and its uses fully explained.

B. NEUROLOGY and PSYCHIATRY

Discussion on:-
1. Trigeminal Neuralgia.
2. Sympathectomy for Peripheral Vascular Disease.
3. Meniere's Syndrome.
4. Raynaud's Disease.
5. Parkinson's Syndrome.
6. Headaches.
7. Vertigo.
8. Nervous Tension.

C. Demonstration and Treatment of Neurological Disease.
1. Insomnia.
2. Parkinson's Disease.
3. Acupuncture Sympathectomy and Treatment of Peripheral Vascular Disease.
4. Meniere's Syndrome.
5. Use of Nervous Tension Points in Ear and Body Acupuncture.
6. Vertigo.

READER'S NOTES

READER'S NOTES

READER'S NOTES

READER'S NOTES